Healthcare Policies in Kazakhstan

Francis E. Amagoh

Healthcare Policies in Kazakhstan

A Public Sector Reform Perspective

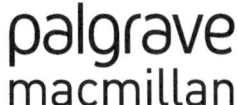

Francis E. Amagoh
Department of Public Administration
KIMEP University
Almaty, Kazakhstan

ISBN 978-981-16-2369-1   ISBN 978-981-16-2370-7   (eBook)
https://doi.org/10.1007/978-981-16-2370-7

This Palgrave Macmillan imprint is published by the registered company Springer Nature Singapore Pte Ltd.
The registered company address is: 152 Beach Road, #21-01/04 Gateway East, Singapore 189721, Singapore

CONTENTS

CONTENTS

LIST OF TABLES

CHAPTER 1

Introduction and Study Background

Access to quality and affordable healthcare constitutes one of the major challenges facing policy-makers in contemporary public administration. Interests abound globally about the need to ensure that health systems meet the needs and demands of citizens, while ensuring efficient and effective use of resources (Amagoh 2011; Analoui 2009; Aringazina et al. 2012). Particularly during periods of fiscal stress, the cost-effectiveness of providing quality and affordable healthcare is of great importance in meeting the needs of populations and safe-guarding their human capital. The effectiveness of a healthcare system is not only measured by the resources utilized, but also by actual outcomes in terms of health indicators (Weale et al. 2016; Tejtivaddhana et al. 2018). As many countries grapple with the ever-increasing costs of healthcare, there have been calls by health experts and international health organizations for major reforms in health systems around the world (Jones et al. 2017; Ministry of Health 2002; Stuart and Lawler 2009). The importance of comprehensive healthcare reforms is particularly relevant in light of the COVID-19 pandemic which has paralyzed the global community since March 2020. While this book does not focus on the responses of the government to the COVID-19 health crisis, it underscores the significance of health systems that are more equipped to respond to pandemic situations. Since its independence on December 16, 1991, Kazakhstan's healthcare system has evolved from centrally controlled and financed, to become more pluralistic and decentralized, where healthcare provider organizations enjoy increased financial

F. E. Amagoh, *Healthcare Policies in Kazakhstan*, https://doi.org/10.1007/978-981-16-2370-7_1

1

and managerial autonomy (Ismailova et al. 2010; Katsaga et al. 2012; Brinkerhoff 2002).

Kazakhstan is one of the countries where multiple reforms in the health sector have been undertaken in an attempt to modernize the *Semashko* model inherited from the Soviet era (Knox 2008; Almagambetova 2011; Kumar et al. 2013). Located in central Asia, Kazakhstan has a unitary form of government, and adopted its first post-Soviet constitution in 1993 (Wilson et al. 2002; Ismailova et al. 2010; Amagoh 2011; Makhmutova 2001), with several amendments made to the constitution starting in October 1998. Kazakhstan has a territory that covers 2,725,000 square kilometers, and is regarded as the ninth largest country in the world in terms of land mass. The country shares borders with China, Russia, Turkmenistan, Uzbekistan, Kyrgyzstan, and part of the Caspian Sea. The size of Kazakhstan's population has increased from 16.45 million in 1991 to 18.864 million in 2020, with a population density of 7 people per square kilometer (18 people per square miles) (Wilson et al. 2002; Knox 2008). Table 1.1 shows some recent demographic information for Kazakhstan.

Administratively, Kazakhstan is comprised of 14 provinces *(oblasts)* and three major cities (Almaty, Nur-Sultan, and Shymkent) (Makhmutova 2001; Perlman and Gleason 2007). The country is governed by an executive President and a legislature that consists of the Senate (Upper House)

Table 1.1 Kazakhstan: Selected recent demographic data

Language	Kazakh is the country's language but Russian is commonly used
Geography	2,725,000 square kilometers
Demographic indicators	
Population	18.867 million (2020)
Population growth rate (%)	0.89 (2020)
Population age 0–14 years (%)	28.9 (2019)
Population age 15–64 years (%)	63.5 (2019)
Population age 65 years and above (%)	7.7 (2019)
Literacy (% of population age 15+)	99.8 (2019)

Sources: (https://knoema.com); Statistical Agency of Kazakhstan (https://stat.gov.kz/); United Nations Educational, Scientific and Cultural Organization (UNESCO) (www.unesco.org); World Bank (www.worldbank.org); Trading Economics (www.tradingeconomics.com/Kazakhstan…); Macro Trends (www.macrotrends.net)

and the *Majilis* (Lower House). The Senate has 49 members who serve 6-year terms. Fifteen of the senators are appointed by the President, while the remaining 34 senators are appointed by *oblast* councils (2 members from each of the 14 *oblasts*, and the three major cities). The Lower House (*Majilis*) has 107 members who serve 5-year terms, based on electoral districts and are elected by popular election. Ninety-eight members of the *Majilis* are directly elected by proportional representation, while 9 members are indirectly elected by *Assembly of People of Kazakhstan* to represent the country's minority population. Aside from cities and towns, Kazakhstan also has villages (*auls*) in rural areas. Each locality elects a local representative body or council (*maslikhat*), known as (*kenes* in the case of *auls*). The elected members of each locality (called deputies) elect a chair (*akim)*. The *akim* is the chief executive of each *oblast* and establishes an administration or *akimat* to manage the delivery of local services (Perlman and Gleason 2007; Wilson et al. 2002; Makhmutova 2001).

1.1   EARLY YEARS OF POLITICAL AND ECONOMIC TRANSITIONS

Kazakhstan faced a series of economic volatility during the early years of independence which were characterized by political and economic transitional challenges (economic liberalization, declining revenues, declining health indicators; government restructuring, policy changes, and funding restrictions) (Ismailova et al. 2010; Shirokova 2007; President of Kazakhstan 1998).

The period of economic turbulence was more pronounced between 1996 and 2007, when the economy would be in a period of growth in some years, only to be followed by periods of economic downturns (World Bank 2010; UNDP 2010; President of Kazakhstan 1997). For example, the economy began to stabilize in 1996, but this was followed by a period of stagnation triggered by the Russian economic crisis in 1998. The economy began to recover in 1999 and accelerated in 2000, largely as a result of the country's booming energy sector. In subsequent years, Kazakhstan's economy enjoyed sustained economic growth with gross domestic product (GDP) growth rates of almost 10% per year, placing the country among the fastest growing economies worldwide (Analoui 2009; World Bank 2010). However, such growth rate was unsustainable, because the extractive sector (mainly oil and gas) accounted for over 70% of the country's exports and about 40% of state revenues. Due to the collapse of commodity prices and the global economic crisis that began in late 2008, Kazakhstan's GDP growth slowed to 3.3% in 2008 but recovered to 7% in 2010 while finally falling back to 4.5% in 2019 (IMF 2014; Committee on Statistics 2020).

Table 1.2 indicates some recent economic indicators for Kazakhstan. In 2019, 4.8% of Kazakhstan's workforce was unemployed, and the Gini index (a measure of social inequality) was 28.8 in 2018. The country experienced a GDP growth of 4.5% in 2019, but this is expected to fall to −2.8% in 2020 due to the COVID-19 pandemic (www.statista.com).

The challenge moving forward is to ensure that subsequent reform policies are sustainable and effective interventions in promoting healthy lifestyles, disease prevention, and pandemic containment (Saner et al. 2008). Total expenditure on health amounted to 3.1% of GDP in Kazakhstan in 2014. Based on latest available figures, the percentages of health expenditure for 2017 and 2018 are 3.1% and 2.92 respectively (www.theglobaleconomy.com).

Kazakhstan derives most of its revenue from oil and gas. While the agricultural sector was estimated to contributed only 4.8% to the GDP in 2017, it is the third largest employer in the country, accounting for 18.1% of the workforce (after the services sector at 61.6% and the industrial sector at 20.4%) (Committee on Statistics 2019).

Table 1.2 Kazakhstan: Selected economic indicators

GDP (billions USD)	181.67 (2019)
GDP growth rate (%)	4.5 (2019)
GDP per capita (USD)	9750 (2019)
Inflation rate (%)	5.2 (2019)
Unemployment rate (%)	4.8 (2019)
Health expenditures as share of GDP (%)	3.1 (2019)
Health expenditure per capita (USD)	280 (2019)
Poverty (% population below national poverty line)	4.2 (2019)
Gini coefficient	28.8 (2018)

Sources: (https://knoema.com); Statistical Agency of Kazakhstan (https://stat.gov.kz/); World Bank (www.worldbank.org); Trading Economics (www.tradingeconomics.com/Kazakhstan…); Macro Trends (www.macrotrends.net)

1.2 Trajectory of Health Indicators

The health system Kazakhstan inherited from the Soviet Union emphasized centralized planning and free universal health coverage for all citizens. While patients had free medical care, there were no choice of doctors, and patients waited in long queues for care, which often led to payment of bribes for better services (Kulzhanov and Rechel 2007). The system did not allow for flexibility that would lead to operational efficiency. Much emphasis was placed on the number of staff and hospital beds, and this created a disincentive for cost-efficiency since such operational aspects of the system were inflated in order to receive more resources from the government (Brinkerhoff and Brinkerhoff 2015). Additionally, the level of funding did not account for quality of care or improved health outcomes (Kuralbaev et al. 2002; World Bank 2007). Table 1.3 shows some governance indicators for Kazakhstan. These indicators have implications for the government's efforts in improving the standards of healthcare for the population.

Table 1.3 Kazakhstan: Selected governance indicators

Corruption perception index (CPI)	34 (2019)
Human development index (HDI)	0.817 (2019)
Rank of the fragile state	59.8 (2020)
Civil society rating	1.2 (2020)
E-government development index	0.8375 (2020)
Press freedom score	52.82 (2019)
Internet users (% of population)	81.88 (2019)

Sources: Freedom House (https://freedomhouse.org); UN Development Program (UNDP) (www.undp.org); Fund for Peace (https://fundforpeace.org/); Transparency International (https://www.transparency.org/en/); United Nations E-government Survey (www.un.org/)

Notes: Civil society ratings are based on a score of 1–7, with lower scores indicating the highest levels of democratic progress. A lower score on the press freedom rankings suggests greater media freedom. The fragile states index scores are from the Fund for Peace website (www.fundforpeace.org). A higher score indicates a more viable state. Civil society ratings and press freedom scores are from Freedom House (www.freedomhouse.org). CPI is from Transparency International website (https://www.transparency.org/en/) The CPI is interpreted as a ranking of countries with scores ranging from 0 (highly corrupt) to 100 (highly clean)

Consequently, Kazakhstan's health system was plagued with poor quality, inefficient services, inequities in the distribution of healthcare resources between urban and rural areas as well as inequities in funding between rural regions and large cities and towns. The government, therefore, realized that healthcare was one of the country's major priorities, and a prerequisite for sustainable development. The country was determined to embark on reforms that would modernize its system of healthcare delivery.

Table 1.4 shows the trend in health indicators from 1990 to 2020 while Table 1.5 shows some recent health indicators. As can be seen from Table 1.4, life expectancy (the number of years a newborn infant is expected to live if the patterns of mortality at the time of its birth were to remain the same throughout its life) for total population increased from 68.3 years in 1990 to 73.9 years in 2020. Infant mortality reduced from 51.4 (per 1000 live births) in 1990 to 9.2 (per 1000 live births) in 2018. Maternal mortality decreased from 78 (per 100,000 live births) in 1990 to 10 (per 100,000 live births) in 2016. Life expectancy for adult males increased from 63.8 years in 1990 to 69.6 years in 2020. A similar positive trend can be observed for adult females. Other positive outcomes brought about by the various health reform programs can be observed from Table 1.4. Table 1.5 shows the most recent available data for some of Kazakhstan's health indicators. According to Kulzhanov and Rechel (2007), the decrease in life expectancy in Kazakhstan in the 1990s and early 2000s was largely due to an increase in deaths from cardiovascular disease, which was common among middle-aged men (OECD 2018; UNESC 2008). Overall mortality from circulatory diseases increased from 598 (per 100, 000 population) in 1990 to 846 (per 100,000 population) in 2005, and decreased to 281.4 (per 100,000 population) in 2015 (Table 1.6). These significant improvements can be attributed to the concerted efforts made by the government of Kazakhstan to improve the country's healthcare system through the various health reform programs.

1.3   CONCLUSION

Kazakhstan emerged from being a member of the former Soviet Union to an independent country that is based on a market economy. At the inception of its independence, the country was confronted with various challenges among which was a healthcare system that was inefficient, ineffective, and incapable of meeting the healthcare needs of the population. Facing the task of building a new nation and modernizing the health system, the government realized the necessity of initiating reform policies

Table 1.4 Some health indicators, 1990–2020 (selected years)

Year	1990	1992	1994	1996	1998	2000	2002	2004	2006	2008	2010	2014	2016	2018	2020
Life expectancy (total population, in years)	68.3	67.7	65.7	64.1	64.6	65.5	65.9	65.9	66.2	67.0	68.3	71.6	72.3	73.2	73.9
Life expectancy at birth, male (in years)	63.8	63	60.6	58.5	59	60.2	60.7	60.4	60.6	61.9	63.5	67.1	68.1	68.8	69.6
Life expectancy at birth, female (in years)	73.1	72.7	71	70	70.4	71.1	71.5	71.7	72	72.4	73.3	75.9	76.6	77.2	78.8
Death rate (per 1000 of population)	8.7	9.3	9.9	10.8	11.2	11.3	11	10.7	10.6	10.4	9.8	8.5	7.4	7.1	7.2
Mortality (per 1000 adult males)	306.3	306.1	364.1	402.1	417.5	410.3	403.1	394	384.1	365.6	336	273	239.6	221.0	–
Mortality (per 1000 adult females)	128.9	147.5	159.7	171.9	175.7	171.2	166.6	161.9	157.1	149.1	137.9	141.2	101.7	94.4	–
Infant mortality (per 1000 live births)	51.4	50.7	49.2	46.4	42.4	37.8	33.5	29.6	26.1	22.6	18.8	11.7	9.8	9.2	–
Under-5 mortality rate (per 1000 live births)	51.8	51.9	52.9	51.7	47.3	42.2	37.3	33.1	28.9	24.7	20.4	13.0	11.0	10.3	10.5
Maternal mortality (per 100,000 live births)	78	80	86	91	81	61	52	46	40	30	22	13	10.0	–	–
Birth rate (per 1000 people)	23.4	21.2	18.9	17.1	15.9	15.6	16.4	18.1	19.9	21.6	22.6	22.6	21.9	21.4	19.9

(continued)

Table 1.4 (continued)

Year	1990	1992	1994	1996	1998	2000	2002	2004	2006	2008	2010	2014	2016	2018	2020
Fertility rate (per woman)	2.83	2.61	2.36	2.13	1.98	1.92	1.99	2.16	2.36	2.54	2.64	2.73	2.73	2.85	2.80

Sources: (https://knoema.com); Statistical Agency of Kazakhstan (https://stat.gov.kz/); United Nations Educational, Scientific and Cultural Organization (UNESCO) (www.unesco.org); World Bank (www.worldbank.org); Trading Economics (www.tradingeconomics.com/Kazakhstan...); Macro Trends (www.macrotrends.net)

Table 1.5 Kazakhstan: selected most recent health indicators

Health indicators	
Infant mortality (per 1000 live births)	7.2 (2020)
Fertility rate (%)	2.7 (2019)
Birth rate (per 1000 population)	16.4 (2020)
Death rate (per 1000 population)	8.2 (2020)
Maternal mortality (per 100,000 live births)	10 (2017)
Neonatal mortality (per 1000 population)	4.7 (2019)
Physicians density (per sq. km)	6.8 (2018)
Hospital bed density (per 1000 population)	6.1 (2014)
Under-5 mortality (per 1000 live births)	10.5 (2019)
Life expectancy total population (years)	73 (2020)
Under-5 years suffering from underweight (%)	2 (2015)
Delivery care coverage (%), skilled attendant at birth	99.4 (2015)
Delivery care coverage (institutional delivery)	99 (2015)
Child malnutrition (% of children under 5 years)	9.3 (2015)

Sources: The World Bank (www.worldbank.org/en/country/kazakhstan); Statistical Agency of Kazakhstan (https://stat.gov.kz/); United Nations Educational, Scientific and Cultural Organization (UNESCO) (www.unesco.org); Ministry of Health of the republic of Kazakhstan (https://www.gov.kz/memleket/entities/); European Observatory on Health Systems and Policies (www.euro.who.int/en/countries/kazakhstan)

Table 1.6 Main causes of death (selected years) (per 100,000 population)

Cause of death	1990	2000	2005	2009	2015
Circulatory diseases	598.0	788.0	846.5	626.4	281.4
Ischemic heart disease	307.3	402.7	381.4	238.5	105.1
Cerebrovascular diseases	202.4	239.6	221.4	180.4	107.4
Infectious diseases	24.1	39.7	31.2	19.4	9.2
Tuberculosis	13.5	30.8	26.4	14.1	4.4
Respiratory diseases	100.8	102.4	81.7	64.6	157.5
Cancer	215.5	190.6	172.2	155.3	125.3
Diseases of the digestive system	38.4	53.1	64.6	58.1	100.1
Mental disorders and diseases of the nervous system	1.6	3.9	4.4	3.1	112.0

Sources: OECD (2018), Kulzhanov and Rechel (2007), Katsaga et al. (2012)

that would address the inadequacies of the healthcare system. This chapter provides an overview of Kazakhstan's political and economic transitions and the trends of the country's healthcare indicators since the early years of independence. The chapter shows that Kazakhstan has made significant improvements in health outcomes since its independence. As will be shown in later chapters of this book, the progress in Kazakhstan's health outcomes has been made possible because of the series of health reform programs instituted by the government, and significant investments in the country's health delivery system.

REFERENCES

Almagambetova, N. (2011). "Kazakhstan primary healthcare: where do the reforms lead us?" Available at: http://www.irex.org/sites/default/files/Nailya A_STG Research Brie….

Amagoh, F. (2011). New public management and healthcare reform in Kazakhstan. *International Journal of Public Administration,* Vol. 34 No. 9, pp. 567–578.

Analoui, F. (2009). Challenges of successful reform: an international perspective. *Journal of Management Development,* Vol. 28 No. 6, pp. 489–494.

Aringazina, A., Gulis, G., and Allegrante, J. (2012). Public health challenges and priorities for Kazakhstan. *Central Asian Journal of Global Health,* Vol. 1 No. 1. Available at: http://cajgh.pitt.edu

Brinkerhoff, D. (2002). Government-nonprofit partners for health sector reform in Central Asia: family group practitioners in Kazakhstan and Kyrgyzstan. *Public Administration and Development,* Vol. 22 No. 1, pp. 51–61.

Brinkerhoff, D. and Brinkerhoff, J. (2015). Public sector management reform in developing countries: perspectives beyond NPM orthodoxy. *Public Administration and Development,* Vol. 35, pp. 222–237.

Committee on Statistics, Ministry of National Economy of the Republic of Kazakhstan. (2019). *Soci-economic Development of the Republic of Kazakhstan,* Nur-Sultan.

Committee on Statistics, Ministry of National Economy of the Republic of Kazakhstan. (2020). *Socio-economic Development of the Republic of Kazakhstan,* Nur-Sultan.

IMF (2014). *Republic of Kazakhstan, Selected Issues,* IMF Country Report No. 14/243.

Ismailova, G., Aydarhanova, K., Demessinov, A. and Aubakirova, A. (2010). Health economic rates for medical services and clinical economic analysis as components of health reform in Kazakhstan. *Medical and Health Sciences Journal,* Vol. 1, pp. 1–7.

Jones, M., Chanturidze, T., Franzen, S., Manu, A., and Naylor, M. (2017). Specifying a state guaranteed health benefits package for Kazakhstan: lessons for emerging economies and middle-income countries. *International Journal of Health Planning Management*, Vol. 32, pp. 540–553.

Katsaga, A., Kulzhanov, M., Karanikolos, M., and Rechel, B. (2012). Kazakhstan: Health system overview. In *Health systems in Transition*, Karanikolos M. and Rechel, B. (eds.), Geneva: European Observatory on Health Systems and Policies.

Knox, C. (2008), "Kazakhstan: Modernizing government in the context of political inertia". *International Review of Administrative Sciences*, Vol. 74 No. 3, pp. 477–496.

Kulzhanov, M., and Rechel, B. (2007). Kazakhstan: Health system overview. In *Health systems in Transition*, B. Rechel (Ed.), Geneva: European Observatory on Health Systems and Policies.

Kumar, A., Izekenova, A. and Abikulova, A. (2013). Inpatient care in Kazakhstan: a comparative analysis. *J Res Med Sci*. Vol. 18, No. 7, pp. 549–553.

Kuralbaev, B., Gavrilova, S., and Kushcanova, Z. (2002). *Forecast of health professionals for the population of Kazakhstan for the period 2003–2010*, Astana, Ministry of Health.

Makhmutova, M. (2001). Local government in Kazakhstan. In Munteanu, I. and Popa, V. (Eds.) *Developing New Rules in Old Environment: Local Government in Eastern Europe, in the Caucasus and in the Central Asia*, The Open Society, Budapest, Chapter 8, pp. 431–447.

Ministry of Health of the Republic of Kazakhstan (2002). *Health of Population and Healthcare of Republic of Kazakhstan, 1991–2001*. Astana, Ministry of Health.

OECD. (2018). *Review of Health Systems: Kazakhstan*. OECD Publishing, Paris.

Perlman, B., and Gleason, G. (2007). Cultural determinism versus administrative logic: Asian values and administrative reform in Kazakhstan and Uzbekistan. *Intl Journal of Public Administration*, Vol. 30, pp. 1–16.

President of Kazakhstan (1997). *Kazakhstan 2030: Prosperity, Security and Welfare for all People of Kazakhstan*. Almaty, President of the Republic of Kazakhstan.

President of Kazakhstan (1998). *The Health of the Nation*, Almaty, President of Republic of Kazakhstan.

Saner, R., Toseva, G., Atamanov, A., and Sahov, A. (2008). Government governance (GG) and inter-ministerial policy coordination (IMPC) in Eastern and Central Europe and Central Asia. *Public Organization Review: A Global Journal*, Vol. 8 No. 3, pp. 215–231.

Shirokova, Y. (2007). Public service standards: international experience, development and implementation in Kazakhstan. *Eurasian Training Center for Civil Servants*, Astana.

statista.com. Kazakhstan: growth rate of the real gross domestic product (GDP) from 2015 to 2025. Available at: www.statista.com/statistics/436121/gross-domestic-product-gdp-growth-rate-in-kazakhstan/

Stuart, N. and Lawler, J. (2009). Managing healthcare under new public management: a sisyphean challenge for nursing. *Journal of Sociology*, Vol. 45 No. 4, pp. 419–432.

theglobaleconomy.com. Kazakhstan: Government spending, percent GDP. Available at: www.theglobaleconomy.com/kazakhstan/government_size/

Tejtivaddhana, P., Briggs, D., Singhadej, O. and Hinoguin, R. (2018). Developing primary healthcare in Thailand: innovation in the use of socioeconomic determinants, sustainable development goals, and the district health strategy. *Public Administration and Policy*, Vol. 21 No. 1, pp. 36–49.

UNDP (2010). *Millennium Development Goals in Kazakhstan*, United Nations Development Program.

UNESC (United Nations Economic and Social Council) (2008). *National Report on the Achievement of Kazakhstan's Strategic Priorities to 2030 in the light of the Millennium Development Goals*. Available at: www.apps01.un.org/nvpcms

Weale, A., Kieslich, K., Littlejohns, P., Tugendhaft, A., Tumilty, E., Weerasuriya, K., and Whitty, J. (2016). Introduction: priority setting, equitable access and public involvement in healthcare. *Journal of Health Organization and Management*, Vol. 30 No. 5, pp. 736–750.

Wilson, J., Gardner, D., Kurganbaeva, G., and Sakharchuk, E. (2002), "The changing role of local government managers in a transitional economy: evidence from the Republic of Kazakhstan", *The International Journal of Public Sector Management*, Vol. 15 No. 5, pp. 399–441.

World Bank (2007). *World Development Indicators.* Washington, DC, World Bank.

World Bank (2010). *Kazakhstan: Data and Statistics.* Available at: www.world-bank.org.kz/website/external/countries/ecaext/kazakhstan

CHAPTER 2

The Need for Health System Design

Healthcare reform has become an important topic of discussion among policy makers and citizens around the globe. Good healthcare is a key driver of human capabilities (Analoui 2009; Gray 2017; WHO 2006) and thus essential to achieving economic and social opportrnities. Good healthcare is to enhance labor productivity, and the provision of healthcare services is expected to optimize people's participation in the economy. Over time, healthcare has increasingly been acknowledged as a key dimension of socio-economic development. Healthcare is at the center of human and economic development and problems in the healthcare system have ripple effects throughout the economy (Kellis and Rumberger 2010; Street and Hakkinen 2009). The healthcare sector in many countries faces complex challenges arising from advances in medical treatment, heightened needs and demands from patients, and decreasing resources to fund healthcare costs (Mirzoev et al. 2007; Sakyi et al. 2011). Several international organizations, such as the World Bank, World Health Organization (WHO), and the Organization for Economic Cooperation and Development (OECD) continue to advise countries (especially developing and transitional economies) on how to design health systems that provide utmost benefits in terms of access, costs, quality, and more choices to citizens. These are attempts to redefine the role of governments in public health governance (Gola 2016; Khayatzadh-Mahani et al. 2013) by ensuring that governments develop policies and take necessary implementation measures that would lead to the desired outcomes. Consequently, the success

F. E. Amagoh, *Healthcare Policies in Kazakhstan*, https://doi.org/10.1007/978-981-16-2370-7_2

of healthcare reform does not only rely on good systems design but also on careful attention to the complex details of implementation (Atun et al. 2007; WHO 2016; World Bank 2014).

Although access has historically been the focus, better health outcomes is also linked to quality improvement measures related to the efficient allocation of resources, and process of delivering healthcare services (that is, health outcomes depend on attributes of performance resulting from the optimization of material inputs and medical practitioner skills). The quantity of healthcare services in terms of material resources, medical staff, medications and infrastructure are prerequisites to achieving inclusive healthcare services (OECD 2018; WHO 2016). The development of healthcare infrastructure, particularly in rural areas, is crucial to enable better access to healthcare services for the poor.

Innovation in healthcare is the key to address the challenges of the twenty-first century in terms of social change and economic sustainability (Habibov 2009; Doskeyeva et al. 2018; Greaves 2017). Designing a world-class healthcare system inevitably requires choosing between or mixing public and private approaches, most particularly in financing. Which choice or mix makes most sense depends in large part on the characteristics of public and private healthcare financing that are feasible. A well-designed health system greatly increases prospects for the success of health programs in terms of health outcomes. This is attained by ensuring adequate provision of resources (money, personnel, information or expertise, physical facilities and equipment, etc.); developing skilled leadership and management capacities that are sensitive to the core of government's mission; and devising institutional arrangements conducive to accomplishing desired objectives (Stabile and Thomson 2014; World Economic Forum 2015; Gray 2017). The complexities of healthcare systems require an appropriate policy framework that integrates the various components of the entire system with significant investments in facilities, technologies, training of health workers, and so on. This means that long-term political commitment is essential for successful healthcare reform policies.

2.1   Goals of Health System Design

Well-designed health systems should ensure increased citizens' access to quality and affordable healthcare either through public sector insurance, private sector insurance, or a combination of both programs. There should be expanded choice of healthcare providers for citizens to choose from.

These should all be targeted to reduce the cost of healthcare for citizens and governments. Access to quality and affordable healthcare and improvements in health status have implications for citizens' quality of life and standard of living, as well as for a country's development (Willis and Khan 2009; Gola 2016; Darisheva et al. 2020; Bolnick 2003). This means improved health outcomes, such as disease reduction and increased life expectancy, reduction in infant and maternal mortality, and so on (Habibov 2009; Atun et al. 2007; UNDP 2010). Since health system has the capacity to significantly contribute to economic development by enhancing the capacity of human capital, governments must pay great attention to its development in terms of organization, regulation, and oversight as an aspect of overall long-term strategy economic development. This is particularly relevant for developing and transitional countries further beset by infrastructural, geographic, and socioeconomic challenges, such as Kazakhstan (Amagoh 2017; Ismailova et al. 2010). Thus, health policies and systems must be designed with a major focus on primary healthcare, which is a prerequisite for achieving the goals of access to care, equity, and improving the wellbeing and health outcomes of citizens (Ibrahim et al. 2011; Katuu 2018; MacLachlan et al. 2012). According to the World Health Organization (Roberts 2009; WHO 2006; Kellis and Rumberger 2010), primary healthcare should be the hub from which patients are guided through the health system.

2.2   Health System's Design Prerequisites

Detailed planning is needed in health system design to prevent waste, make full use of scare resources, contain costs to what is affordable, and ensure that they are distributed geographically on an equitable basis. This is essential for a vastly large country like Kazakhstan. This means that effective health system design requires substantive and governance reforms (Smith and Nguyen 2013; President of Kazakhstan 2017).

Substantive healthcare reform entails purposive changes in the structure and organization of the health system. On the other hand, governance healthcare reform emphasizes changes in the management, leadership, configuration and jurisdiction of different actors in the health system.

Substantive reforms emphasizes the reform of certain aspects of the structure and organization of health services, but do not necessarily aim to make significant changes to governance arrangements. Efforts aimed to improving the health system through introduction of clinical networks (Pham 2011; Tam et al. 2018; Weale et al. 2016) and improvements in patient safety through individual diligence (UNDP 2010; World Economic Forum 2015; WHO 2006) are good examples of substantive reforms. It should be noted here that if the system in which individuals operate is not receptive to changes called for in the reform, it can be difficult for individual diligence to have an impact (Essen 2009; Knox 2008; Tejtivaddhana et al. 2018). This is where governance reform is also necessary in order to effect change.

Governance reform deals with changing how health systems are governed, and the relationships between the various actors in the system. It is concerned with the division of control and patterns of interaction among key actors in the system. This is because the organization of health systems varies across multiple dimensions, such as public versus market; roles and responsibilities for central, regional and local public institutions; and different forms of interactions between public institutions and the market at these levels (Lynn 2006; Sakyi et al. 2011). Designing governance is a process that caters to a multitude of objectives. It must accommodate basic ideas about representation and accountability and secure the capabilities to get things done. Government actors and institutions must therefore forge coalitions with key actors in their external environment. Designing governance is about facilitating effective representation and accountability (Witesman and Wise 2009; Smith and Nguyen 2013). Consequently, when policies dictate market solutions to solve public policy issues, governance is adapted to facilitate such change by empowering the bureaucracy and other levels of government.

2.3   Functions of Health System's Structure

Healthcare systems must perform various functions designed to achieve measurable objectives. To work effectively, a healthcare system must perform three basic functions, namely, *delivering services, creating resources,* and *financing* (Bolnick 2003; Stabile and Thomson 2014). Delivering services is the function that is most felt by the citizens. It is this function that has a direct impact on the population. However, in order to deliver services, the health system must first be effective at creating resources needed to deliver the services. This can be done through investment in physical and human capital as well as training of healthcare workers. Funds are needed to ensure that the functions of service delivery and resource creation are met. This means that health systems must also arrange the necessary financing needed to achieve the objectives of the health system. Economic activities of financing, creating resources, and delivering services might take place in either the public or private sectors or a mix of both (Bolnick 2003; Gola 2016; Nonkhuntodd and Yu 2018).

The World Health Organization has three fundamental objectives of how health systems should perform, namely, improvement of the health of the population served; responsiveness to citizen's expectations of their "needs" and "wants"; and financial fairness in providing protection against the costs of poor health. It is therefore imperative that health systems be designed with the aim of reaching these objectives (WHO 2016; Mirzoev and Kane 2018).

It should be noted that it is impossible to have a world-class health system without the long-term commitment of the legislative and executive branches of government. This means that there should be enlightened regulation and policies on how to ensure that universal access to medical care is attainable to all citizens. Whether totally public, totally private or mixed public–private healthcare systems, thee should be enlightened commitment and stewardship of governments in order to achieve a desirable long-term sustainable health system. Additionally, the healthcare system must be flexible and able to adapt to new healthcare technologies and new medical care needs. As medical research continues to drive new breakthroughs in innovation and technology, citizens will begin to value more cutting-edge medical care (Bolnick 2003; Atun et al. 2007; Gola 2016).

2.4   Conclusion

Successful health systems' outcomes depend on an optimal system design and stringent implementation with efficient allocation of resources. It requires appropriate long-term policy frameworks that allow for seamless implementation of designed systems. Optimal healthcare systems must ensure access to quality and affordable healthcare for all citizens through some sort of health insurance (public, private, or a combination of both) and the freedom of citizens to choose their healthcare providers.

To be successful, health system' design should incorporate features of substantive and governance reforms that emphasize changes in the health delivery system and the relationship between all the actors in the system. It is only when these two features of reform are included in health system design that the system can achieve its objectives.

REFERENCES

Amagoh, F. (2017). Healthcare in Kazakhstan. In *The Future of Healthcare in Developing Countries in Asia*. C. Asplata and K. Pribadi (eds.). Routledge, London.

Analoui, F. (2009). Challenges of successful reform: an international perspective. *Journal of Management Development*, Vol. 28 No. 6, pp. 489–494.

Atun, R., Kyratsis, I., Jelic, G., Rados-Malicbegovic, D., and Gurol-Urganci, I. (2007). Diffusion of complex health innovations: Implementation of primary healthcare reforms in Bosnia and Herzegovina. *Health Policy and Planning*, Vol. 22, pp. 28–39.

Bolnick, H. (2003). Designing a world-class health system. *North American Actuarial Journal*, Vol. 7 No. 2, pp. 1–23.

Darisheva, M., Tracy, M., Terlikbayeva, A., Zhussupov, B., Schluger, N. and McCrimmon, T. (2020). Knowledge and attitudes toward ambulatory treatment of tuberculosis in Kazakhstan. *BMC Health Services Research*, Vol. 20, pp. 1–10.

Doskeyeva, G., Rakhimbekova, A., Zhambeyeva, M., Saudambekova, I., and Bekova, R. (2018). Health care financing system in the Republic of Kazakhstan. *European Research Studies Journal*, Vol. XXI No. 2, pp. 282–288.

Essen, A. (2009). New hospital payment systems: Comparing medical strategies in The Netherlands, Germany and England. *Journal of Health Organizations and Management*, Vol. 23 No. 3, pp. 304–318.

Gola, S. (2016). Medical tourism in India: whose interest? *Journal of International Trade Law and Policy*, Vol. 15 No. 2/3, pp. 115–133.

Gray, M. (2017). Population healthcare: designing population-based systems. *Journal of the Royal Society of Medicine*, Vol. 10 No. 5, pp. 183–187.

Greaves, D. (2017). Evidence-based management of Caribbean health systems: barriers and opportunities. *International Journal of Health Governance*, Vol. 22 No. 2, pp. 104–117.

Habibov, N. (2009). Determinants of out-of-pocket expenditures on prescribed medications in Tajikistan: Implications for healthcare sector reform. *Journal of Health, Organization and Management*, Vol. 23 No. 2, pp. 170–182.

Ibrahim, Y., Khan, M., and Khan, J. (2011). An assessment of the performance of reform in Nigeria and Malaysian national health scheme program. *International Journal of Business and Social Science*, Vol. 2 No. 21, pp. 145–156.

Ismailova, G., Aydarhanova, K., Demessinov, A. and Aubakirova, A. (2010). Health economic rates for medical services and clinical economic analysis as components of health reform in Kazakhstan. *Medical and Health Sciences Journal*, Vol. 1, pp. 1–7.

Katuu, S. (2018). Healthcare systems: typologies, framework, models and South Africa's health sector. *International Journal of Health Governance*, Vol. 23 No. 2, pp. 134–148.

Kellis, D., and Rumberger, J. (2010). Health reform and the hospital industry: what can we expect?, *Journal of Healthcare Management*, Vol. 55 No. 4, pp. 283–296.

Khayatzadh-Mahani, A., Nekoei-Moghdam, M., Esfandiari, A., Ramezani, F. and Parva, S. (2013). Clinical governance implementation: a developing country perspective. *Clinical Governance: An International Journal*, Vol. 18 No. 3, pp. 186–199.

Knox, C. (2008). Kazakhstan: Modernizing government in the context of political inertia. *International Review of Administrative Sciences*, Vol. 74 No. 3, 477–496.

Lynn, L. (2006). *Public Management: Old and New*. Abingdon: Routledge.

MacLachlan, M., Khasnabis, C. and Mannan, H. (2012). Inclusive health. *Tropical Medicine and International Health*, Vol. 17, No. 1, pp. 139–141.

Mirzoev, T., and Kane, S. (2018). Key strategies to improve systems for managing patient complaints within health facilities: What can we learn from existing literature? *Global Health Action*, Vol. 11 No. 1, pp. 1–14.

Mirzoev, T., Green, A., and Newell, J. (2007). Progress towards health reform in Tajikistan. *Journal of Health Organization and Management*, Vol. 21 No. 6, pp. 495–505.

Nonkhuntodd, R. and Yu S. (2018). Lessons from Thailand: universal healthcare achievements and challenges. *International Journal of Social Economics*, Vol. 45 No. 2, pp. 387–401.

OECD. (2018). *Review of Health Systems: Kazakhstan*. OECD Publishing, Paris.

Pham, T. (2011). Efficiency and productivity in hospitals in Vietnam. *Journal of Health Organization and Management*, Vol. 25 No. 2, pp. 195–213.

The President of Kazakhstan Nursultan Nazarbayev's Address to the Nation of Kazakhstan on January 31, 2017, Third Modernization of Kazakhstan: Global Competitiveness. Available at: http://www.akorda.kz/en/addresses/addresses_of_president/the-president-of-kazakhstan-nursultan-nazarbayevs-address-to-the-nation-of-kazakhstan-january-31-2017

Roberts, A. (2009). The politics of healthcare reform in post-communist Europe: the importance of access. *Int. Publ. Pol.*, Vol. 29 No. 3, pp. 305–325.

Sakyi, E., Awoonor-Williams, J. and Adzei, F. (2011). Barriers to implementing health sector administrative decentralization in Ghana: a study of the Nkwanta district health management team. *Journal of Health Organization and Management*, Vol. 25 No. 2, pp. 400–419.

Smith, O and Nguyen, S. N (2013). *Getting Better: Improving Health System Outcomes in Europe and Central Asia*. Europe and Central Asia Reports. Washington, DC: World Bank Group. Available at: http://documents.worldbank.org/curated/en/953751468250295078/Getting-betterimproving-health-system-outcomes-in-Europe-and-Central-Asia

Stabile, M and S. Thomson (2014). The changing role of government in financing health care: an international perspective. *Journal of Economic Literature*, Vol 52 No. 2, pp. 480–518.

Street, A. and Hakkinen, U. (2009). Health system productivity and efficiency", in Smith P.C. et al. (eds.), *Performance Measurement for Health System Improvement. Experiences, Challenges and Prospects*, Cambridge University Press, New York (on behalf of European Observatory on Health Systems and Policies), pp. 222–248.

Tam, T., Tran, T., Prueksaritanond, S., Isidro, J., Setia, S. and Welluppilai, V. (2018). Integrated health care systems in Asia: an urgent necessity. *Dove Press*. Available at: file:///C:/Users/famagoh/Des top/Healthcare%20in%20 KZ%20Book_Literature/Integrated%20health%20care%20systems%20in%20 Asia%20an%20urgent%20necessity%20CIA.htm

Tejtivaddhana, P., Briggs, D., Singhadej, O. and Hinoguin, R. (2018). Developing primary healthcare in Thailand: innovation in the use of socioeconomic determinants, sustainable development goals, and the district health strategy. *Public Administration and Policy*, Vol. 21 No. 1, pp. 36–49.

UNDP (United Nations Development Program) (2010). The real wealth of nations: pathways to human development. Available at: www.undp.kz/en/articles/1/75.jsp

Weale, A., Kieslich, K., Littlejohns, P., Tugendhaft, A., Tumilty, E., Weerasuriya, K., and Whitty, J. (2016). Introduction: priority setting, equitable access and public involvement in healthcare. *Journal of Health Organization and Management*, Vol. 30 No. 5, pp. 736–750.

Willis, K. and Khan, S. (2009). Health reform in Latin America and Africa: decentralization, participation and inequalities. *Third World Quarterly*, Vol. 30 No. 5, pp. 991–1005.

Witesman, E. and Wise, C. (2009). The centralization/decentralization paradox in civil service reform: how government structure affects democratic training of civil servants. *Public Administration Review*, Vol. 69 No.1, pp. 116–127.

World Bank. (2014). *Universal Health Coverage for Inclusive and Sustainable Development. A Synthesis of 11 Country Case Studies*. Directions in Development. Human Development. Washington, DC.

World Economic Forum. (2015). *Benchmarking Inclusive Growth and Development*. World Economic Forum Discussion Paper. January.

World Health Organization (WHO). (2006). *The World Health Report 2006. Working Together for Health*. WHO, Geneva.

WHO (2016). *Integrated Care models: An overview*. WHO Regional Office for Europe, Copenhagen.

CHAPTER 3

Overview of Kazakhstan's Health System

A health system is comprised of several constitutive parts. Such parts include primary healthcare, inpatient care, outpatient care, hospital care, and so on (Gray 2017; Bolnick 2003; Doskeyeva et al. 2018). Since its independence in 1991, Kazakhstan has launched several health reform programs aimed at improving its health system through increased access, granting more autonomy to healthcare institutions, and reducing reliance on inpatient care. However, the health system still has some of the vestiges of a transitional economy undergoing restructuring (OECD 2018a; Ismailova et al. 2010; Aringazina et al. 2012; Birtanov 2016). The reforms have led to a reorganization of the system in which the Ministry of Health plays a prominent role. Kazakhstan inherited a Semashko model of healthcare with excessive centralization of health functions at the center. Health service delivery continues to undergo various reforms with tangible evidence to indicate progress in the health system. During the Soviet era, there was limited role for primary healthcare. Health promotion was limited, and services were delivered through hospitals based on disease or population criteria (Amagoh 2011; Kumar et al. 2013). Healthcare facilities were owned and centrally managed by the government. The task before a newly independent Kazakhstan was therefore to redesign the health system in ways that incorporate western standards, with the view to achieving positive health outcomes through health system modernization. This meant revitalizing primary care, encouraging private practice, and granting autonomy to health providers. As one of the fundamental

© The Author(s), under exclusive license to Springer Nature Singapore Pte Ltd. 2021
F. E. Amagoh, *Healthcare Policies in Kazakhstan*,
https://doi.org/10.1007/978-981-16-2370-7_3

components of a health system, the next section will discuss the progress Kazakhstan has made in primary healthcare.

3.1   PRIMARY HEALTHCARE

According to the World Health Organization, primary healthcare is a whole-of-society approach to health and wellbeing with a focus on the health needs of individuals, families, and communities. It addresses the general determinants of health and the comprehensive and interrelated aspects of physical, mental, and social health and wellbeing (WHO 2016; Analoui 2009; OECD 2016). After independence, Kazakhstan's primary healthcare had significant fragmentation which impeded effective health service delivery.

To build effective primary healthcare system, countries should invest more in the key functions of primary care and less on costly inpatient facilities (Gray 2017; Jones et al. 2017; Kulzhanov and Rechel 2007). This means primary healthcare structures, which act as first points of contact for patients within the health system, must be effective and efficient enough to coordinate patient care, and offer referrals to specialists in secondary healthcare when necessary. Kazakhstan is devoting significant attention to the modernization of its primary healthcare. This development of primary healthcare services in Kazakhstan began after its independence even though the country, while part of the Soviet Union, was where the 1978 Declaration of the Alma-Ata (the first major international conference highlighting the central role of primary healthcare in health systems) was hosted (Ministry of Health 2011; Brinkerhoff 2002). Efforts toward implementing a primary healthcare system only became evident after the country became independent. These efforts have been sustained, and the primary healthcare system in Kazakhstan has considerably improved.

3.2   ELEMENTS OF PRIMARY HEALTHCARE
IN KAZAKHSTAN

A number of activities are considered as part of the primary healthcare. These activities are as follows:

(i) Diagnosis for early detection of diseases;
(ii) Treatment on an outpatient basis;
(iii) Inpatient care (i.e., day hospital, hospital at home);

(iv)   Examination of temporary disability;
(v)   Preventive examinations;
(vi)   Immunization;
(vii) Promotion of healthy lifestyles;
(viii) Recommendations on rational and healthy eating;
(ix)   Family planning;
(x)   Maternity and childbirth services;
(xi)   Monitoring of health status; and
(xii) Implementing free screening (Ministry of Health 2016; Katsaga et al. 2012).

3.3   RESPONSIBLE ENTITIES AND PROGRAMS

A number of entities are tasked with various aspects of primary healthcare in Kazakhstan. They include the following:

1. *National Centre for Problems of Healthy Lifestyle Development:* This body is responsible for the establishment of the list of non-communicable diseases based on population needs. It is also responsible for providing training and other broader public health functions.

2. *National Screening Program:* Established by the government in 2008, the aim of this program is to address the strategic objectives in the fight against non-communicable diseases in the country.

3. *National Center for Problems of Healthy Lifestyle Development:* Established in 1997, the aim was to oversee the implementation of the country's overarching development strategy *(Kazakhstan 2030)* which aimed to make Kazakhstan one of the 30 most advanced economies by 2030. This entity coordinates all analysis, monitoring, evaluation, and reporting on the implementation of the *National Screening Program.* The mission of the center is the development and implementation of all national policies related to healthy lifestyle development in Kazakhstan. Some of its activities include:

   (i) The implementation and governance mechanisms of healthy lifestyle programs and prevention of diseases;
   (ii) Liaising with ministries, agencies, and local authorities in the implementation of health promotion programs;

(iii) Ensuring the development and deployment of new technologies to improve the health of the various population groups;

(iv) Training of primary healthcare and healthy lifestyle professionals, health educators on disease prevention, health promotion and healthy lifestyles; and

(v) Engaging with various population groups and the media to develop and promote healthy lifestyle principles. (OECD 2018a; Kulzhanov and Rechel 2007).

4. *Department for the Organization of Medical Services:* Located under the Ministry of Health, this is the main body responsible for designing and monitoring the implementation of primary healthcare policies in Kazakhstan.

5. *Medical Services Standardization Department:* The main responsibility of the department is the drafting and coordination of medical protocols and managing certain aspects of primary healthcare facilities (such as organizing the training of healthcare managers).

6. *Observatory of Human Resources for Health:* This entity develops all policies related to human resources in the health sector and coordinates their deployment across the country.

7. *National Center for Problems in Healthy Lifestyle Development:* This center has the major responsibility of developing and implementing national healthy lifestyle policies that are partly implemented by primary healthcare facilities in Kazakhstan.

8. *Committee for the Protection of Public Health* and the *Department of Strategy Development in Public Health:* Since 2017, these two bodies have oversight responsibilities for all activities concerning infectious diseases surveillance. Health authorities at local levels are responsible for implementing state level policies and organizing the provision of healthcare and responsibly monitoring the performance of facilities. (Ministry of Health 2016; OECD 2018a).

The number of primary healthcare facilities in Kazakhstan was estimated to be about 6280 in 2015 though some of them are ill-equipped, with most of them located in rural areas (Ministry of Health 2016; WHO 2015).

3.4   Categories of Primary Healthcare Staff

While there are physicians who have the main task of taking care of the healthcare needs of primary healthcare patients, there are also a number of other categories of workers in the primary healthcare system. These include:

- *Primary healthcare nurses.* They generally work with physicians, and their responsibilities include the provision of nursing care in health facilities, or in the residence of patients during home visits. Primary healthcare nurses also evaluate the health status of patients and give advice on disease prevention.
- *Midwives.* This category of staff is responsible for clinical and administrative tasks, such as keeping medical records, performing pregnancy tests, providing antenatal care, and providing assistance with deliveries during pregnancies.
- *Feldshers.* These are mid-level career staff common in most former Soviet countries. They usually provide emergency care in rural facilities, but can also provide consultations and prepare patients for medical examinations (Katsaga et al. 2012; World Bank 2010; UNDP 2011).
- *Social workers and psychologists* are also involved in primary healthcare services. They provide social and psychological support to patients either in outpatient or home settings (OECD 2018a).

3.5   Categories of Primary Healthcare Facilities

Primary healthcare facilities in urban areas were granted more autonomy in their operations in the early 2000s when polyclinics in urban areas were legally separated from hospitals (Ismailova et al. 2010; WHO 2011). This move gave them more independence in managing resources. However, rural primary healthcare facilities (such as feldsher-midwifery posts and physician ambulatories) are still administratively part of central rayon hospitals. In addition to primary healthcare facilities engaging in private practice, there are five categories of government facilities: *government institutions; state enterprises; state enterprises with the right of economic management;* and *joint stock companies.*

- *Government institutions*: Public healthcare facilities in this category do not have the autonomy to manage their own budgets or fixed assets, as they are entirely under the control of the Ministry of Health or local health authority. They provide services entirely as defined by the government. Usually, they treat socially significant diseases, such as tuberculosis or they are psychiatric hospitals.
- *State enterprises*: These are institutions that can independently manage their own budget, but under certain conditions, since they are still under some control of the Ministry of Health. They are also allowed to charge fees for services; however, staff remunerations (such as salaries and bonus) are established by the Ministry of Health or the local health authority. They are financed according to contracts with a single-payer, or on the basis of the services provided (such as hospitals or outpatient clinics). They can also be financed on a capitation basis as in the case of primary healthcare providers.
- *State enterprises with right of economic management*: Healthcare institutions in this category are the most autonomous of the public healthcare providers. They independently manage their budgets, and can open branches and representative offices across the country. However, they need the approval of the Ministry of Health or local health authority in order to set the prices of the services provided. Supervisory boards to oversee their activities were established in 2011. These boards are responsible for their management and financial governance. They are now the most common status of healthcare facilities. While they have autonomy to manage the revenues of the facility, parts of the proceeds of the operations are shared with the state. For example, a staff payroll ceiling is defined by the Ministry of Health or local health authority, while the salaries and bonuses are managed by the facility. However, the Ministry of Health or local health authority is responsible for the salaries of the CEO, deputies, and chief accountant of the facility.
- *Joint Stock Companies* (JSC): Ownership of such facilities is held by shareholders and subject to state law. They are financed through contracts with a single-payer. A good example is the fact that in 2011 the National Medical Holding became a joint stock company which incorporates six national medical centers and the Astana Medical University under a single management authority. However, most of the staffs contracted are not considered as civil servants.

- *Private Facilities Providing State Guaranteed Benefit Package*: These are fully private facilities with the aim of providing services through the private market, but were given an exceptional right to provide services through the State Guaranteed Benefits Package. (Ministry of Health 2015; OECD 2018a).

3.6   THE HOSPITAL SECTOR

There has also been increased autonomy granted to hospitals in Kazakhstan, a far departure from what was practiced during the Soviet era. This includes more autonomy in the operations of public facilities, payments based on diagnostic-related diseases, accreditation of facilities, and the development of specialized services (Birtanov 2016; IMF 2017; Kuralbaev et al. 2002; Kumar et al. 2013; Katsaga et al. 2012; OECD 2018b).

3.6.1   Major Categories of Hospital Facilities

There are six categories of hospital facilities in Kazakhstan, as described below.

1. *Rural hospitals:* These institutions are the foundation of rural inpatient care in Kazakhstan. Rural hospitals usually are located in small towns and villages and are small health facilities with about 20–25 beds. They are mostly devoted to basic emergency and secondary care as well as maternity and outpatient care. These remote facilities are also involved in patient referral and transportation services.
2. *Rayon hospitals:* These are hospital facilities that are somewhat larger in capacity than rural hospitals. They are usually located in the largest towns in each *rayon*, and typically have between 100 and 300 beds. They have a range of healthcare specialists and various advanced diagnostic equipment. They also play referral roles for patients with severe medical conditions that need more complex care.
3. *Secondary multi-profile hospitals:* These are much larger hospital facilities located in the major town of an *oblast*. They have extensive capacity and can accommodate between 600 and 1000 beds. These hospitals offer a variety of specialized care and use more modern and state-of-the-art technology.
4. *Tertiary hospitals:* These are also called National (Republican) hospitals. These are hospital facilities that provide highly specialized

care to patients. They are involved in conducting research and coordinating national health programs. They also serve as clinical teaching facilities for medical students and are located mostly in Almaty and Nur-Sultan. They include research institutions for cancer, obstetrics, gynecology, psychiatry, and so on. There are 8 high-level tertiary health institutes in Kazakhstan as listed below.

- Healthcare Development Institute;
- National Institute of Cardiology and Internal Diseases;
- National Research Center for Mother and Child Health;
- National Children's Rehabilitation Centre;
- National Diagnostic Center;
- Scientific Center of Neurosurgery;
- Scientific Research Institute of Emergency Care; and
- National Research Cardiac Surgery Center.

5. *Polyclinics:* Health institutions in this category can either be freestanding or located in hospitals as outpatient units. They offer a range of primary and secondary care services. Even when located in a hospital facility, polyclinics have their own manager and staff and operate independently from the hospital system. A significant number of polyclinics in Kazakhstan are state-owned and have beds that can be used for inpatient or outpatient care.

6. *Mono-profile hospitals:* As in most former Soviet countries, mono-profile hospitals are part of the hospital system. They are numerous in number and are established to provide care for specific disease or population groups (such as tuberculosis, psychiatric conditions, maternal and child health, sexually transmitted diseases, other infectious diseases, addiction disorders, and hospice services). Most the disease conditions treated in mono-profile hospitals can be treated in outpatient facilities or in some of the other categories of hospitals discussed above.

Other information about the hospital system show that as at 2015, the number of hospital beds per capita in Kazakhstan was 4.8 per 1000 people, with mono-profile facilities representing 40% of the bed capacity. The mix of public to private hospitals in Kazakhstan had also increased. For example, between 1999 and 2004, the number of private facilities almost tripled. In 1999, 10% of all physicians were working in the private sector;

by 2010 this share had increased to 16% (Ministry of Health 2011). By 2011, 16.4% of all physicians in Kazakhstan were working in the private sector. In 2012, the state owned 777 hospitals while 136 hospitals were privately owned (Kumar et al. 2013: Ministry of Health 2016).

3.7   HOSPITAL MODERNIZATION INITIATIVES

At the beginning of its independence in 1991, Kazakhstan had 740 publicly owned hospitals. This number grew to 895 in 2006, with more diverse ownership, mostly resulting from decentralization (WHO 2011; Kulzhanov and Rechel 2007; Ministry of Health 2011). The 1995 *Law of Self-Government* introduced a series of new legal statuses under which public facilities can operate. Subsequent reforms expanded the authority of the Ministry of Health and introduced a new regulatory environment, with greater health system centralization and financing functions (Makhmutova 2001; Amagoh 2011; Brinkerhoff 2002). The authorities initiated the strengthening and modernization of the hospital sector with targeted investments and reorganization. This includes modernizing the regulatory environment with a consolidated health budget at national level, while public providers are given more autonomy (Shrokova 2007; Jones et al. 2017; Kulzhanov and Rechel 2007). In addition, private provision of hospital services has been encouraged with the aim of fostering competition in health service delivery. To support this, a number of initiatives were established to enhance quality assurance and to direct patients' choice of hospital facilities.

3.8   OTHER ASPECTS OF THE HEALTH SYSTEM

1. *Pharmaceutical care:* The reforms have also focused on developing the pharmaceutical industry. Since 2000, there has been a rapid increase in the pharmaceutical market with Kazakhstan becoming one of the major pharmaceutical markets in countries of the former Soviet Union (Amagoh 2011; Aringazina et al. 2012; Doskeyeva et al. 2018). For example, in 2008 the turnover of pharmaceuticals in Kazakhstan accounted for 0.1% of global pharmaceutical market (Ismailova et al. 2010; Jones et al. 2017). In the same year, the shares of domestic producers constituted 10% of consumed pharmaceuticals while 90% of were imported. In 2010, there were 9990

pharmacy organizations in Kazakhstan. This consisted of 6572 pharmacies, 844 pharmacy posts, 1184 pharmacy kiosks, and 1390 pharmaceutical warehouses (Ministry of Health 2011; OECD 2018b).

2. *Rehabilitation and long-term care:* Efforts are being made to modernize rehabilitation and long-term care. These efforts are coordinated by the Ministry of Health, the Ministry of Labor and Social Protection, as well as the Ministry of Education. Active role is also being played by a number with of NGOs in this regard. Most notable NGOs that assist the government in rehabilitation and long-term care include the *National Research and Practice Center of Social Adaptation* and *Professional Rehabilitation of Children and Adolescents with Developmental Deficiencies* which provides medical and social assistance to children with developmental deficiencies. The costs are covered from the *oblast* or republican health budgets, depending on the administrative level of the provider (World Bank 2010; WHO 2015).

3. *Palliative care:* According to the *Code on People's Health and the Healthcare System* of 1993, the following provisions are made for palliative care: first, palliative care can be provided under the guidance of physicians to terminally ill patients in the final stage of their lives. Such care should be taken in specialized units of independent medical organizations (hospices) or in their homes; second, palliative care may be provided by qualified nurses when guidance by physicians in such specialized units, independent organizations (nursing homes), or patients' homes are not required (President of Kazakhstan 2009; WHO 2015).

4. *Mental healthcare:* Government Resolution No. 468 of 30 March 2000 guarantees access to mental healthcare. This includes diagnosis, treatment, and rehabilitation. Psychiatric problems are included in the list of "hazardous diseases" defined by *Government Resolution* and mental health patients are eligible for free-of-charge outpatient pharmaceuticals (Katsaga et al. 2012; Aringazina et al. 2012; Amagoh 2011; Almagambetova 2011). The *Code on People's Health and the Healthcare System* identifies certain criteria for psychiatric care. This includes:

- methods for providing voluntary and compulsory referrals for people with psychiatric disorder;
- guidelines on how to restrict people with psychiatric disorders when under the care of health professionals;

- guaranteed rights for people with psychiatric care;
- the process of diagnosing and treatment of people with psychiatric disorders;
- mechanism of psychiatric care and social protection are delivered by the state;
- procedures to be followed during the process of hospitalization and discharge;
- measures to ensure safety of psychiatric patients. (President of Kazakhstan 2009; Ministry of Health 2011).

5. *Dental healthcare:* The health reforms have also facilitated the emergence of a significant number of private practice in dental healthcare. Most dental care in Kazakhstan is now provided in the private sector. These dental clinics, including some that are government-owned, are well equipped with state-of-the-art dental technologies and most of them are located in Almaty and Nur-Sultan. However, access to quality dental healthcare services is still poor in rural areas. All dental products imported into the country must be registered with the Ministry of Health. After being registered, the products are entered into the *List of Medical Products, Registered and Permitted for Medical Use in the Territory of Republic of Kazakhstan.* The registration is valid for 3–5 years after which it must be renewed (UNESC 2008; Committee on Statistics 2016).

6. *Health Promotion:* As part of the reforms, health promotion activities were included in the State Guaranteed Benefits Package. Coordination committees were established at national and regional levels to ensure that the public is informed on various aspects of healthy lifestyle. The healthy lifestyles service includes teachers and healthcare specialists providing services and counselling to children and adolescents about healthy living. Other health professionals focus on information about exercise and healthy diets. The *National Centre for Healthy Lifestyles* collaborates with *oblast* and city health departments to increase the role and capacity of primary healthcare in health promotion. They focus on such issues as the prevention of alcohol and tobacco consumption; drug abuse; chronic and communicable diseases; sexually transmitted infections and HIV/AIDS; accidents and poisonings; promotion of physical activity; healthy nutrition; and reproductive health (Ministry of Health 2011; OECD 2018a, b).

3.9   Conclusion

Primary healthcare and the hospital system constitute important elements of focus in any healthcare modernization plan. As primary healthcare focuses on the health and wellbeing of individuals, families, and communities, it is the foundation of the health and human capital of societies. Similarly, hospitals and health clinics are the major mechanisms through which health services are delivered to citizens. This chapter examined the primary healthcare and hospital system that form the foundation of Kazakhstan's healthcare system. The chapter examined the various transformations that have occurred in the health system since the country gained its independence. The various modernization initiatives and innovations that have occurred in Kazakhstan's health system are due to the numerous health reform initiatives of the government. These transformations are also evident in other aspects of the health system, such as pharmaceutical care, dental care, and promotion of health lifestyles. The implementation of these initiatives is made possible by the structural reorganization of the health system, as is discussed in Chap. 4.

References

Almagambetova, N. (2011). Kazakhstan primary healthcare: where do the reforms lead us? Available at: http://www.irex.org/sites/default/files/Nailya A_STG Research Brie…

Amagoh, F. (2011). New public management and healthcare reform in Kazakhstan. *International Journal of Public Administration,* Vol. 34 No. 9, pp. 567–578.

Analoui, F. (2009). Challenges of successful reform: an international perspective. *Journal of Management Development,* Vol. 28 No. 6, pp. 489–494.

Aringazina, A., Gulis, G., and Allegrante, J. (2012). Public health challenges and priorities for Kazakhstan. *Central Asian Journal of Global Health,* Vol. 1 No. 1. Available at: http://cajgh.pitt.edu

Birtanov, Y. (2016), Kazakhstan gears up to launch social health insurance. *Bulletin of the World Health Organization.* Volume 94, pp. 792–793

Bolnick, H. (2003). Designing a world-class health system. *North American Actuarial Journal,* Vol. 7 No. 2, pp. 1–23.

Brinkerhoff, D. (2002). Government-nonprofit partners for health sector reform in Central Asia: family group practitioners in Kazakhstan and Kyrgyzstan. *Public Administration and Development,* Vol. 22 No. 1, pp. 51–61.

Committee on Statistics, Ministry of National Economy of the Republic Kazakhstan (2016), *Socio-economic development of the Republic of Kazakhstan,* Astana.

Doskeyeva, G., Rakhimbekova, A., Zhambeyeva, M., Saudambekova, I., and Bekova, R. (2018). Health care financing system in the Republic of Kazakhstan. *European Research Studies Journal,* Vol. XXI No. 2, pp. 282–288.

Gray, M. (2017). Population healthcare: designing population-based systems. *Journal of the Royal Society of Medicine,* Vol. 10 No. 5, pp. 183–187.

IMF (2017), World Economic Outlook Database.

Ismailova, G., Aydarhanova, K., Demessinov, A. and Aubakirova, A. (2010). Health economic rates for medical services and clinical economic analysis as components of health reform in Kazakhstan. *Medical and Health Sciences Journal,* Vol. 1, pp. 1–7.

Jones, M., Chanturidze, T., Franzen, S., Manu, A., and Naylor, M. (2017). Specifying a state guaranteed health benefits package for Kazakhstan: lessons for emerging economies and middle-income countries, *International Journal of Planning Management,* Vol. 32, pp. 540–553.

Katsaga, A., Kulzhanov, M., Karanikolos, M., and Rechel, B. (2012). Kazakhstan: Health system overview. *In Health systems in Transition,* Karanikolos M. and Rechel, B. (eds.), Geneva: European Observatory on Health Systems and Policies.

Kuralbaev, B., Gavrilova, S. and Kuschanova, Z. (2002). Forecast of health professionals provision for the population of Kazakhstan for the period 2003–2010. Astana, Ministry of Health.

Kulzhanov, M. and Rechel, B. (2007). "Kazakhstan: Health system overview" *In Health systems in Transition,* B. Rechel (Ed.), Geneva: European Observatory on Health Systems and Policies.

Kumar, A., Izekenova, A. and Abikulova, A. (2013). Inpatient care in Kazakhstan: A comparative analysis. *J Res Med Sci.* Vol. 18, No. 7, pp. 549–553. http://www.ncbi.nlm.nih.gov/pmc/articles/PMC3897019

Makhmutova, M. (2001). Local government in Kazakhstan. In Munteanu, I. and Popa, V. (Eds.) *Developing New Rules in Old Environment: Local Government in Eastern Europe, in the Caucasus and in the Central Asia,* The Open Society, Budapest, Chapter 8, pp. 431–447.

Ministry of Health. (2011). Health of the population of the Republic of Kazakhstan and performance of health organizations. Astana.

Ministry of Health. (2015). National health accounts of the Republic of Kazakhstan. A report on health care expenditure for the year 2014.

Ministry of Health. (2016). Population health in the Republic of Kazakhstan and activity of health care Organizations in 2015, Kazakhstan.

OECD (2017), *Caring for Quality in Health: Lessons learnt from 15 reviews of healthcare quality,* OECD Publishing, Paris.

OECD. (2018a). *Review of Health Systems: Kazakhstan.* OECD Publishing, Paris.

OECD (2018b). *National Health Accounts of Kazakhstan,* OECD Publishing, Paris. Available at: https://doi.org/10.1787/9789264289604-en

OECD (2016). *Multi-dimensional Review of Kazakhstan: Volume 1. Initial Assessment*, OECD Publishing, Paris. Available at: https://doi.org/10.1787/9789264246768-en

President of Kazakhstan (2009). *Code on People's Health and the Healthcare System.* Presidential Decree No. 193-IV. Almaty, President of the Republic of Kazakhstan.

Shrokova, Y. (2007), Public service standards: international experience, development and implementation in Kazakhstan. *Eurasian Training Center for Civil Servants*, Astana.

UNESC (United Nations Economic and Social Council). (2008). *National report on the achievement of Kazakhstan's strategic priorities to 2030 in the light of the Millennium Development Goals.* United Nations.

UNDP (United Nations Development Program). (2011). National human development report for Kazakhstan. United Nations.

World Bank. (2010). *Kazakhstan: Data and Statistics.* World Bank.

WHO (World Health Organization). (2011). *Evaluation of the organization and provision of primary care in Kazakhstan – a survey-based project in the regions of Almaty and Zhambyl,* World Health Organization, Geneva.

WHO (World Health Organization). (2015). *Ambulatory care sensitive conditions in Kazakhstan.* World Health Organization, Geneva.

WHO (World Health Organization). (2016). *Integrated care models: an overview.* WHO Regional Office for Europe, Copenhagen.

CHAPTER 4

Organization of the Health Delivery System

The structure of Kazakhstan's health system has evolved from initially being a rayon-level system with strict subordination to the national level, to subsequently an *oblast*-level system with greater autonomy, and currently a system where hospital and primary healthcare are divided between the national and *oblast* levels (Dikanbayeva 2010; Aringazina et al. 2012; Makhmutova 2001). The health delivery system is structured in a way that gives the Ministry of Health the central organizing authority of the health system. Since its independence in 1991, Kazakhstan's national health policies are set by the national government and implemented by national and local authorities (Kulzhanov and Rechel 2007; Amagoh 2011; Knox 2008). In the past, public health was hierarchically organized, and most public health service provisions had centralized monitoring, inspection, and mandatory sanitary services. The reforms have reduced the degree of centralization by giving more powers to regional and local authorities (Ismailova et al. 2010; Wilson et al. 2002; UNDP 2012). This means that authorities at the *oblast, rayon*, and *city* levels have specified responsibilities.

Typically, rural policlinics are generally staffed by four types of physicians: adult therapist, pediatrician, obstetrician, and stomatologist (dentist). Smaller rural hospitals with about 20–30 beds offer very limited treatment. At the *rayon* level, each *rayon* has a central town hospital that offers basic care. These hospitals also have ambulatory policlinics staffed by medical specialists. The main city in the *oblast* has specialist hospitals and specialized dispensaries for long-term conditions, such as tuberculosis

© The Author(s), under exclusive license to Springer Nature   35
Singapore Pte Ltd. 2021
F. E. Amagoh, *Healthcare Policies in Kazakhstan*,
https://doi.org/10.1007/978-981-16-2370-7_4

and cancer (WHO 2011; OECD 2018a; UNDP 2016). The central health authority is responsible for certain hospitals in major cities like Almaty and Nur Sultan, which provide advanced and specialist treatments for conditions such as cardiovascular diseases and cancer. The central health authority is also responsible for sanitary epidemiological services (Saniped or SES) which focus on environmental surveillance and control of communicable diseases (Birtanov 2016; UNDP 2016; Ministry of Health 2011).

4.1   HEALTH DELIVERY STRUCTURE

4.1.1   *Ministry of Health*

As part of a wider public sector reform in Kazakhstan, the organizational structure of the Ministry of Health has undergone several changes since Kazakhstan gained its independence in 1991 with various name changes as follows.

- Initially it was called the *Ministry of Health* in 1991;
- It was later renamed the *Committee of Health* within the *Ministry of Education, Culture and Health* in 1997.
- In 1999, the *Committee of Health* was renamed the *Agency of Health*.
- It was finally renamed the *Ministry of Health* in 2002. (Ministry of Health 2004; Katsaga et al. 2012).

These transformations were all associated with management changes in the overall healthcare system. The Ministry of Health is at the apex of the health system's hierarchy, while services are administered mainly by *oblast* (regional) departments, which have considerable autonomy in running health services in their respective areas.

The Ministry of Health has the main functions of formulating health policies, and regulating and coordinating the relationships within the various agencies, and between the health system and other sectors in the economy (Ministry of Health 2015; OECD 2018a; World Bank 2018). Furthermore, the Ministry of Health sometimes performs service delivery functions through national clinical centers.

Itemized functions of the Ministry of Health as stipulated in the *Code on People's Health and the Healthcare System* of 2009 include:

- Implementation of health policies at the national level;

- Developing innovative health planning systems;
- Approving delivery arrangements for health services;
- Developing healthcare legislation and regulations;
- Development and approval of healthcare standards;
- Monitoring and evaluation of healthcare organizations;
- Organizing continuous education, training and retraining of medical and pharmaceutical staff;
- Appointments of heads of local health administrations;
- Developing agreements with heads of local executive bodies on programs for achieving performance targets;
- Development and facilitating inter-sectoral cooperation;
- Regulating prices of drugs and medical services provided by state health organizations;
- Purchase of health services within the State Guaranteed Benefits Package, in line with budget programs;
- Accreditation of healthcare entities;
- Coordinating with NGOs about the implementation of national health policies;
- Supervision of the activities of health entities;
- Developing the list of drugs and medical supplies purchased from a single distributor responsible for procuring and supplying drugs and medical supplies; and
- Ensuring the preparedness of organizations responsible for the prevention and management of emergency situations. (Kulzhanov and Rechel 2007; Ministry of Health 2015)

4.1.2   Committees under the Ministry of Health

The Ministry of Health has three subordinate committees that help to implement health policies in the regions and at national level. They are: *Committee of Pharmacy*, *Health Services Purchasing Committee (KOMU)*; and *Committee for the Protection of Public Health*. These three committees have representations in all *oblasts*, and the chairpersons of the Committees report to the Minister of Health at the national level. The Committees have the following main tasks:

- *Committee of Pharmacy:* This Committee is responsible for quality assurance and control. It oversees issues such as accreditation, licensing, and certification of entities involved in the provision of healthcare services. It is also responsible for quality audits and the investigation of patient complaints.

- *Health Services Purchasing Committee (known as KOMU):* This Committee purchases all publicly funded health services through contractual arrangements. It is responsible for health financing arrangements. Some of its objectives include: establishing a "level playing field" between public and private players, and reducing disparities in funding between regions.
- *Committee for the Protection of Public Health:* The main responsibility of this committee is the implementation of policies regarding matters of sanitary and epidemiological wellbeing of the population. It has oversight on public health and sanitary-epidemiological services. This includes prevention and control of infectious diseases; monitoring of sanitary-epidemiological conditions, quality of water and food items, and monitoring of laboratory safety. (Ministry of Health 2015; OECD 2018a; Katsaga et al. 2012)

4.2   Oblast Health Departments (Also Known as Local Health Authorities)

Health departments at *oblast* level are located in all the 15 regions in the country and the cities of Almaty and Nur-Sultan. They are responsible for managing healthcare delivery and own most of the healthcare facilities in their respective jurisdictions.

However, they have no control over National Clinics, Research Centers, and University hospitals, which are owned by the Ministry of Health (OECD 2018a).

Oblast health departments are part of *oblast* administrations. The directors of *oblast* health departments are appointed by the *oblast akims* (governors) to whom they are accountable, in coordination with the Ministry of Health. The *Oblasts* manage all state-owned healthcare providers in their jurisdictions, and the directors of *oblast* health departments have the authority to appoint and dismiss the heads of health organizations, and supervise their activities (Ministry of Health 2009; UNDP 2019). Key functions of *oblast* health departments are as follows:

- Implementation of a single-payer function within *oblasts* (as long as this has not been pooled at national level);

- Planning of health expenditure within local budgets;
- Contracting and paying healthcare providers;
- Control of the expenditures of state-owned healthcare providers;
- Establishing and maintaining the unified health information system at the *oblast* level; and
- Appointing and dismissing the heads of state-owned health organizations in their territory. (Ministry of Health 2011; OECD 2018a)

With regard to healthcare functions, *oblast* administrative bodies (*akimats* and *maslihats*) have the following responsibilities:

- Ensuring that residents' rights to the State Guaranteed Benefits Package, in compliance with established state standards are realized;
- Appointing and dismissing the heads of *oblast* health departments;
- Planning and approval of local expenditures according to health program budgets;
- Implementing inter-sectoral collaboration in the area of health protection; and
- Making decisions on the establishment of state-owned health facilities. (Ministry of Health 2009, 2015; OECD 2018b)

It should be noted that *rayons* do not have any financial authority. Their responsibility is only limited to transporting ambulatory patients to health service providers (OECD 2018b; Ministry of Health 2002; UNDP 2019).

4.3   HEALTH FINANCING

Financing of healthcare has been one of the core instruments used to reform the operations and instill professionalism in Kazakhstan's health system. The *Ministry of Economic Affairs and Budget Planning* and the *Ministry of Finance* regulate health financing mechanisms and allocate the health budget.

The Ministry of Health has a *Finance Department* that is responsible for the financing of medical education and capital investments in Kazakhstan. It is also responsible for certain components of the State Guaranteed Benefits Program. This includes, for instance, reimbursement of health providers at the national level (e.g., the Republican Psychiatric Hospital, Leprosarium, AIDS Centre, etc.) and sanitary aviation. It also finances treatments for "socially significant" diseases (such as, cancer, tuberculosis, etc.). All of these activities are financed either through direct payments to healthcare providers or through designated allocations to the Oblast Health Departments.

In addition, the *Health Services Purchasing Committee (KOMU)* finances a significant part of the State Guaranteed Benefits Program, such as:

1. Inpatient care treated within urban multi-profile hospitals, which are reimbursed and fall under three categories: specialized care, day care, and tertiary care. Inpatient care for socially significant diseases (such as tuberculosis, psychiatry/substance abuse, infectious diseases, HIV/AIDS, oncology) is excluded from this funding system; and
2. It is responsible for the financing of ambulatory care in urban and areas, and rural areas as well as cancer care. (OECD 2018a; Katsaga et al. 2012; World Bank 2018).

Table 4.1 shows Kazakhstan's health expenditure from 2000 to 2017. Total health expenditures as percentage of GDP decreased from 4.16% in 2000 to 3.13% in 2017. Similar decreases can be found in government health expenditure as percentage of GDP which decreased from 2.12% in

Table 4.1   Kazakhstan health expenditure data 2000–2017 (selected years)

Health expenditure	*2000*	*2002*	*2004*	*2006*	*2008*	*2010*	*2012*	*2014*	*2016*	*2017*
Total health expenditure as % of GDP	4.16	3.61	3.98	3.40	3.05	2.74	3.06	2.71	3.43	3.13
Government health expenditure as % of GDP	2.12	1.93	2.32	2.31	2.27	1.87	2.07	1.87	2.06	1.94
Government health expenditure as % of total budget	9.25	9.42	10.91	11.69	8.37	8.32	9.45	8.79	9.59	7.87
Government health expenditure per capita (USD)	26	32	65	119	189	169	254	237	157	174

Sources: Ministry of Health (2015); World Bank (www.worldbank.org); (www.countryeconomy.com/...); (www.macrotrends.net/...); (www.tradingeconomics.com/...)

2000 to 1.94% in 2017. Government health expenditure as percentage of total budget also decreased from 9.25% in 2000 to 7.87% in 2017. Remarkably, there was a significant increase in government health expenditure per capita (USD) from 26USD in 2000 to 174USD in 2017.

One of the main focuses of the reforms was the modernization of primary healthcare in the country. In line with reform efforts, financial allocation to primary healthcare increased in subsequent years. For example, in 2005, primary healthcare received 28% of the total health budget; an increase from an estimated share of 10% in the mid-1990s. By 2010, the primary healthcare sector accounted for at least 40% of public healthcare resources allocated for the implementation of the state-guaranteed package of services (Ministry of Health 2004). Primary healthcare expenditure as percentage of the total healthcare budget also increased from 25% in 2018 to 40% in 2019 (Satubaldina 2018; World Bank 2018; Prime Minister of Kazakhstan 2019).

4.4   The Urban/Rural Divide

While inequities in healthcare delivery still exist between the urban and rural areas in Kazakhstan, the health reforms have reduced this gap. Urban areas have better-equipped facilities and healthcare staff. Urban areas have polyclinics, which are large medical facilities to provide both primary and secondary ambulatory care. Such medical facilities have about 20 medical specialties, as well as diagnostic and laboratory services (Ministry of Health 2015; WHO 2011; Katsaga et al. 2012).

This is in contrast to rural areas where healthcare organizations lack adequate personnel and advanced medical facilities. The inequities were so serious that in 1999, more than 1200 villages and small settlements had no resident healthcare facilities. In response, the government in 1999 enacted the *Decree on Measures for Improving Primary Healthcare for the Rural Population*. This measure established minimum standards for the public provision of rural health services (Ministry of Health 2002; World Bank 2004; UNDP 2004).

Healthcare services in rural areas are provided by rural physician ambulatories, *feldsher*-midwifery posts (FAPs) and medical posts. Physicians in rural clinics receive referrals from the *feldsher*-midwifery posts and provide basic healthcare services. The FAPs are staffed with *feldshers* (lower level medical professionals), physician assistants, and/or midwives. During the Soviet era, the FAPs were the first point of contact with health professionals for the rural population. The staff provided simple curative, antenatal, and postnatal care while actual deliveries were referred to the nearest hospital. They also undertook basic disease prevention activities such as immunization and health education, and dispensed medication prescribed by doctors.

As part of the reforms in the health system, the Ministry of Health in 2006 introduced much larger medical posts that provide a wider range of services in rural areas. Other problems in rural areas include a lack of adequate transportation between dispersed villages and the central town of the district where there are large hospitals. To address this problem, the Ministry of Health developed a system of telemedicine which enables medical specialists to organize long-distance conferences for diagnosis and counselling. By 2010, telemedicine had been introduced in all the *oblasts* of the country.

4.5   Conclusion

The structural reorganization of Kazakhstan's health system, while giving the Ministry of Health the central role of developing health policies for Kazakhstan, provides regional and local authorities more responsibilities on how healthcare services are delivered to citizens. The itemized functions of the Ministry of Health and oblast authorities are aimed at eliminating duplications and redundancies in the health system and provide measure of accountability for each line of authority and responsibility.

A major concern for the Ministry of Health is reducing the inequities in healthcare delivery between urban and rural areas of Kazakhstan. While these inequities have been considerably alleviated, subsequent healthcare reforms are expected to reduce them much further.

References

Amagoh, F. (2011). New public management and healthcare reform in Kazakhstan. *International Journal of Public Administration,* Vol. 34 No. 9, pp. 567–578.

Aringazina, A., Gulis, G., and Allegrante, J. (2012). Public health challenges and priorities for Kazakhstan. *Central Asian Journal of Global Health,* Vol. 1 No. 1. Available at: http://cajgh.pitt.edu

Birtanov, Y. (2016). Kazakhstan gears up to launch social health insurance. *Bulletin of the World Health Organization.* Volume 94, pp. 792–793

Dikanbayeva, S. (2010). *Health lifestyles development policy: policy and management in the Republic of Kazakhstan.* Astana, National Center for Healthy Lifestyles.

Ismailova, G., Aydarhanova, K., Demessinov, A. and Aubakirova, A. (2010). Health economic rates for medical services and clinical economic analysis as components of health reform in Kazakhstan. *Medical and Health Sciences Journal,* Vol. 1, pp. 1–7.

Katsaga, A., Kulzhanov, M., Karanikolos, M., and Rechel, B. (2012). Kazakhstan: Health system overview. *In Health systems in Transition,* Karanikolos M. and Rechel, B. (eds.), Geneva: European Observatory on Health Systems and Policies.

Knox, C. (2008). Kazakhstan: modernizing government in the context of political inertia. *International Review of Administrative Sciences,* Vol. 74 No. 3, pp. 477–496.

Kulzhanov, M., and Rechel, B. (2007). Kazakhstan: health system overview. *In Health systems in Transition,* B. Rechel (Ed.), Geneva: European Observatory on Health Systems and Policies.

Makhmutova, M. (2001). Local government in Kazakhstan. In Munteanu, I. and Popa, V. (Eds.) *Developing New Rules in Old Environment: Local Government in Eastern Europe, in the Caucasus and in the Central Asia,* The Open Society, Budapest, Chapter 8, pp. 431–447.

Ministry of Health of the Republic of Kazakhstan. (2002), *Health of Population and Healthcare of Republic of Kazakhstan, 1991–2001.* Astana, Ministry of Health.

Ministry of Health of the Republic of Kazakhstan. (2004). *National Program of Health Reform and Development for 2005–2010. Approved by Presidential Decree on 13 September, 2004.* Astana, Ministry of Health.

Ministry of Health. (2009). Health of the population of the Republic of Kazakhstan and performance of health organization in 2008 (statistical collection). Astana.

Ministry of Health. (2011). Health of the population of the Republic of Kazakhstan and performance of health organizations. Astana.

MOH (2015). *Population Health in the Republic of Kazakhstan and Activity of health care organizations in 2014,* Kazakhstan.

OECD. (2018a). *Review of Health Systems: Kazakhstan.* OECD Publishing, Paris.

OECD (2018b). *National Health Accounts of Kazakhstan.* OECD Publishing, Paris. https://doi.org/10.1787/9789264289604-en.

Prime Minister of Kazakhstan. (2019). *Emphasis on Healthy Lifestyles and Human Capital: About the Program of Healthcare Development 2020–2025.* Nur-Sultan, Kazakhstan.

Satubaldina, A. (2018). Kazakhstan gears up primary healthcare coverage. Available at: https://astanatimes.com/2018/09/kazakhstan-gears-up-primary-healthcare-coverage/#:~:text=As%20part%20of%20the%20national,21%20percent%20and%20increase%20the

UNDP (United Nations Development Program). (2004). Human development report Kazakhstan 2004. Education for all: the key goal for a new millennium. UNDP, New York.

UNDP (United Nations Development Program). (2012). The real wealth of nations: pathways to human development. UNDP, New York.

UNDP (United Nations Development Program) (2016). National human development report for Kazakhstan: sustainable development goals and capability based development in regions of Kazakhstan. UNDP, New York.

UNDP (United Nations Development Program) (2019). National human development report for Kazakhstan: urbanization as an accelerator of inclusive and sustainable development. UNDP, New York.

Wilson, J., Gardner, D., Kurganbaeva, G., and Sakharchuk, E. (2002). The changing role of local government managers in a transitional economy: evidence from the Republic of Kazakhstan. *The International Journal of Public Sector Management,* Vol. 15 No.5, pp. 399–441.

(The) World Bank (2004). Comments on the National Program of Health Sector Reform and Development in the Republic of Kazakhstan for 2005–2010. Washington, DC, World Bank.

(The) World Bank. (2018). *World Development Indicators.* Washington, DC. World Bank.

WHO (2011). *Evaluation of the Organization and Provision of Primary Care in Kazakhstan – A survey-based project in the regions of Almaty and Zhambyl,* World Health Organization, Geneva.

CHAPTER 5

Trajectory of Health Reforms

The provision of health services in Kazakhstan has evolved from the *Semashko* model of the Soviet system which emphasized mostly on hospital services and neglected the importance of primary healthcare, disease prevention, and health promotion (Ministry of Health 2016). Several healthcare reforms have been made over the years with the aim of making the government more responsive and effective in meeting the health challenges of the population. These reforms are part of the public sector reform movement which aims to make government more efficient in delivering public services in a cost-effective manner (Katsaga et al. 2012; Pavlovskaya 2013). As a form of continuous improvement, Kazakhstan has enacted healthcare reform policies every few years since its independence. These health reform policies are examined in this chapter.

5.1   The Concept of Healthcare Reform (1992)

The first comprehensive move for health reform in post-Soviet Kazakhstan was in 1992 when it enacted *The Concept of Healthcare Reform*. As a country that had just gained its independence, and with an awareness of the failings of the Soviet model, Kazakhstan was willing to initiate the process of healthcare modernization. Among the main features of the *Concept of Healthcare Reform* are the following:

F. E. Amagoh, *Healthcare Policies in Kazakhstan*, https://doi.org/10.1007/978-981-16-2370-7_5

A. Establishment of a health insurance scheme: Aimed to ensure that all citizens were insured for basic healthcare coverage, which was one of the features of the Soviet model;

B. Decentralization of health administration: The goal of decentralization of health administration was to ensure that the responsibilities for healthcare delivery were devolved to regional and local governments which are closer to the people in order to have a more effective and efficient delivery of health services.

C. Reduction of hospital beds: High hospital occupancy was one the characteristics of the Soviet health system. Hospital administrators were rewarded based on how many hospital beds were occupied. This led to high inefficiencies since it discouraged outpatient services. Consequently, this reform was to reduce hospital costs borne by the government by ensuring that only patients with severe medical conditions were admitted as inpatients in the hospitals.

D. A focus on primary healthcare: This element was lacking in the Soviet healthcare system which focused less on disease prevention and more on hospital services. Newly independent Kazakhstan realized that primary healthcare is the foundation for a healthy population. As a result, this provision was included in the new reform to provide necessary preventive care and all necessary health screenings.

E. The right to private practice for healthcare professionals: Contrary to the practice during the Soviet Union, this provision allowed health professionals to have private healthcare facilities as long as they met all required professional standards under the law. This was also needed to promote competition in the healthcare system.

F. Patient's right to choose a doctor: During the Soviet era, patients were assigned a doctor by the government. This provision in the health reform gave citizens the right to choose their own doctors. This was also needed to enhance competition between public and private healthcare providers.

G. Improved training for healthcare professionals: Modernization of the health system could not be achieved without retraining of healthcare professionals based on western best practices. The government realized that as a country that was in the process of transition, this was one of the prerequisites needed for upgrading the healthcare delivery system in the country. (Ministry of Health 2002; Kulzhanov and Rechel 2007)

5.2   MANDATORY HEALTH INSURANCE (1996)

In 1996, a Mandatory Health Insurance Fund was introduced to be funded through payroll tax whereby employers deducted 3% of workers' salaries towards the insurance fund. *Oblast* administrations were responsible for paying such fees for socially vulnerable groups, while self-employed individuals had to pay for their own insurance. This program was unsuccessful nationwide and was abandoned in 1998. Since 1999, the national budget became the single public source of healthcare financing (Ministry of Health 2011; Committee on Statistics 2016).

5.3   THE PRESIDENT'S "STRATEGY KAZAKHSTAN 2030" (1997)

In 1997, the President announced *Strategy Kazakhstan 2030* which included healthcare as one of the policy imperatives for the development of the country (President of Kazakhstan, 1997). The health policy goals in the strategy include the following:

- development of a healthy lifestyle;
- health promotion programs across the country;
- emphasis on disease prevention;
- primary healthcare, and so on. (Ministry of Health, 2002)

As part of its efforts to improve the health of the population, in 1997 the government established the *National Center for Healthy Lifestyles.* The aim was to develop strategies that encourage healthy lifestyles among the population.

The *National Center* was established to aid in the implementation of the country's development strategy, *Kazakhstan 2030.* The mission of the *National Center* is the development and implementation of national policies related to healthy lifestyle development in Kazakhstan. Among its key activities are the following: (a) implementation and governance of healthy lifestyle programs and disease prevention; (b) collaboration with agencies and local authorities in the implementation of health promotion programs; (c) training of primary healthcare and healthy lifestyle professionals and educators on disease prevention, health promotion, and healthy lifestyles; and (d) collaboration with population groups and the media to promote healthy lifestyle principles (National Center for Healthy Lifestyle 2016; Kulzhanov and Rechel 2007).

5.4   Law on the Health of the Nation (1998)

The government established the *Law on the Health of the Nation* 1998. The law was rather broad and provided a comprehensive review of the health issues facing the country (such as modernization, infrastructural challenges, training of healthcare workers, etc.). The law developed broad strategies and goals aimed at addressing the challenges by the end of 2008 (Ministry of Health 2011).

5.5   Decree on Measures for Improving Primary Healthcare for the Rural Population (1999)

Due to the inequities in the delivery of health services in rural areas, the President issued the *Decree on Measures for Improving Primary Heath Care for the Rural Population*. The purpose of the decree was to establish minimum standards for the public provision of rural healthcare services. These standards were meant to be reviewed and improved periodically to meet the challenges of healthcare delivery in rural parts of the country (Ministry of Health 2002, 2011).

5.6   National Program for Healthcare Reform and Development 2005–2010 (2004)

In 2004, the government of Kazakhstan enacted the *National Program for Healthcare Reform and Development for 2005–2010*. This was part of a broader development strategy called *"Towards a Competitive Kazakhstan, a Competitive Economy and a Competitive Nation"*. This healthcare reform program was perhaps the most comprehensive health reform effort that Kazakhstan had undertaken at that time. The government realized that a robust healthcare program was a prerequisite for developing the country's human capital and ensuring a competitive economy in the global community (Ministry of Health 2004; Kulzhanov and Rechel 2007; Katsaga et al. 2012).

As stipulated in the *National Program for Healthcare Reform and Development for 2005–2010*, the aim of the program was to improve the quality of health service provision; develop a new regulatory framework for the healthcare system; ensure equitable access to health services; and significantly move towards primary and outpatient care. A number of policy priorities were identified to be addressed by the end of 2010. These priority tasks include the following:

- a shift towards primary healthcare;
- a shift from inpatient to outpatient care;
- using international best practices in healthcare delivery;
- the use of new technologies, advanced treatment methods, and medical services;
- improvements in maternal and child health;
- training of health professionals and health managers;
- prevention, diagnosis and treatment of "socially significant diseases"; and
- improvements in the physical infrastructure (buildings, equipment, etc.) of health facilities. (Ministry of Health 2004)

This health reform program also introduced a state-guaranteed basic benefits package of services (such as, emergency care, outpatient care and inpatient care) free of charge for citizens and paid from the national budget. User fees were only allowed for services outside the basic benefits package. Under this healthcare reform program, the *Concept on the Unified Healthcare System* was established in 2009 with the aim of improving transparency and competition in the health system.

5.7   State Healthcare Development Program for 2011–2015 (Salamaty Kazakhstan) (2010)

The *State Healthcare Development Program*, also called *Salamaty Kazakhstan* was adopted in 2010. Implementation of the program was rolled out in phases from 2011 to 2015. *Salamaty Kazakhstan* had much emphasis on the following:

- Improving public healthy lifestyles;
- Developing quality domestic pharmaceutical industry;
- Improving the accessibility and quality of primary healthcare;
- Developing mechanisms to reduce inpatient care;

- Reallocating more resources to primary healthcare and disease prevention;
- Improving benefit plans for health workers, particularly in rural areas;
- Enhancing training standards for medical staff;
- Increasing the capacity of human resources;
- Improving palliative care; and
- Enhancing gerontological and geriatric services. (President of Kazakhstan 2010)

Salamaty Kazakhstan also aimed to improve rehabilitation and long-term care, especially through the establishment of a network of rehabilitation facilities and outpatient hospitals. It established several benchmarks on which to measure the success of the reform program. These include:

- An increase of 50% in the share of domestic drug manufacturing by 2015.
- Increase in life expectancy to 69.5 years by 2013, and 70 years by 2015;
- Decrease in total mortality rate to 8.14 per 1000 by 2013, and 7.62 per 1000 by 2015;
- Decrease in maternal mortality rate to 28.1 per 100,000 by 2013, and 24.5 per 100,000 by 2015; and
- Decrease in infant mortality rate to 14.1 per 1000 by 2013 and 12.3 per 1000 by 2015 (Ministry of Health 2011; Almagambetova 2011).

5.8   STATE POLICY FOR PUBLIC HEALTH DEVELOPMENT 2016–2019 (DENSAULYK) (2015)

In 2015, the government enacted the *State Policy for Public Health Development for 2016–2019* (also called Densaulyk).The main goal of the reform policy is to ensure the development of an effective and sustainable system that would protect the health of the population. Features of this healthcare reform policy include:

- Empowering and educating the population in health promotion and disease prevention. This includes measures to avoid exposure to environmental, dietary, and behavioral risks;
- Improving surveillance of communicable and non-communicable diseases;

- Improving measures to prevent and assess mental health disorders, road safety, and injury prevention;
- Improving communication channels between the state, private sector, and non-governmental organizations;
- Strengthening public health legislation and regulation;
- Optimizing long-term disease modeling to better forecast risks at the regional and national levels;
- Upgrading medical and pharmaceutical education to be in line with western standards; and
- Improving quality of, and accessibility to, public health programs. (Ministry of Health 2015; OECD 2018)

Densaulyk requires that at regional levels, the development, planning, implementation, and monitoring of disease prevention activities would be conducted in collaboration with primary healthcare facilities, including screening and preventive medical examinations. Special emphasis would be placed on prevention and monitoring of the main burden of diseases in Kazakhstan (cardiovascular diseases, injuries, cancer, tuberculosis, diabetes) (WHO 2016; World Bank 2018).

An important priority area of focus is health workforce training with emphasis on the *European Program of Core Competences for Public Health Professionals*, which defines the range of competencies for public health professionals. This is meant to advance and reinforce the competencies of healthcare professionals. Currently in Kazakhstan, public health education is offered at bachelor degree level, through post-master's and doctoral degree (PhD) programs. There are also continuing professional education (CPE) courses that provide supplementary, advanced, and updated training for health professionals (Committee on Statistics 2016; Ministry of Health 2018).

5.9 State Program of Healthcare Development 2020–2025 (2019)

In December 2019, the government of Kazakhstan passed the most recent health reform program: the *State Program of Healthcare Development 2020–2025*.

The reform is aimed at placing more focus on healthy lifestyle and improved public health services. It also targets improvement in the quality of medical services and a sustainable development of the health system. Other elements in the reform include the following:

- An increase in people's choice for quality health services;
- Modernization of public health services;
- Provision of comprehensive primary healthcare;
- Healthcare as a factor in human capital development;
- Improving medical care delivery system;
- Creating a single digital healthcare space;
- Implementation of compulsory health insurance and promotion of voluntary health insurance to achieve universal health coverage;
- Improving investment opportunities in the medical industry; and
- Good governance in healthcare (Ministry of Health 2020; President of Kazakhstan 2020).

Kazakhstan, through this reform will take steps to become member of the *International Council for Harmonization of Technical Requirements for Pharmaceuticals for Human Use (ICH)* and *the Medical Device Regulators Forum (IMDRF)*. The reform also aims to have a substantial renewal of regional healthcare infrastructure through a program to build modern hospitals of international standards through public–private partnerships. In this effort, development centers of best practice in the area of primary healthcare will be strengthened with advance technologies. Kazakhstan's major healthcare reform milestones are shown on Table 5.1.

5.10   Conclusion

The *Semashko* health model which Kazakhstan inherited from the Soviet Union was proven to be ineffective and inefficient. The various health reform policies that Kazakhstan has undertaken over the years are efforts to address the myriad of healthcare challenges that the country inherited from the Soviet Union after its independence. These reforms are attempts to ensure optimal and modern health service for the population, and the government of Kazakhstan has been commended for such efforts by international organizations (World Bank 2004; WHO 2011).

The most recent health reform policy (State Program of Healthcare Development 2020–2025) which was passed in 2019 did not anticipate the COVID-19 pandemic and as result, measures on how to respond to pandemic situations were not considered. As Kazakhstan has been able to

Table 5.1 Kazakhstan's healthcare reform milestones

Year	Health reforms adopted and their features
1992	*The Concept on Healthcare Reform* adopted. It called for: mandatory health insurance; an increased role for primary healthcare; decentralization of administration; establishment of private practice; patients' right to choose healthcare providers; improved training for health professionals
1996	*Mandatory Health Insurance Fund* (MHIF) with payroll tax funding introduced but abandoned in 1998
1997	The President's *Strategy Kazakhstan 2030* which sets out broad social policy agenda for the country. This includes health policy goals, such as the development of healthy lifestyles and other areas of health promotion and disease prevention
1998	The *Law on the Health of the Nation* was adopted. It provided an in-depth review of health issues in the country. Strategies and broad goals were established with ways to achieve them by 2008
1999	*Decree on Measures for Improving Primary Healthcare for the Rural Population* was adopted to establish minimum standards for provision of rural health services and reduce some of the challenges of health provision in rural parts of the country
2004	The *National Program for Healthcare Reform and Development 2005–2010* was adopted. This program was implemented from 2005 to 2010. The aim was to improve the quality and efficiency of health services; create a new regulatory framework; ensure equitable access to health services; achieve a shift towards primary and outpatient care; etc.
2010	Adoption of the *State Healthcare Development Program for 2011–2015 (Salamaty Kazakhstan)*. This program was implemented from 2011 to 2015 with goals such as, improving public healthy lifestyles; developing quality domestic pharmaceutical industry; improving the accessibility and quality of primary healthcare; develop mechanisms to reduce inpatient care; reallocate more resources to primary healthcare and disease prevention; etc.
2015	*State Policy for Public Health 2016–2019 (Densaulyq)* focused on developing a modern and sustainable health system with emphasis on disease prevention; training and education of healthcare workers; etc.
2019	*State Program of Healthcare Development 2020–2025* emphasizes healthy lifestyles and improvement in the quality of healthcare services improved primary healthcare services; compulsory health insurance; etc.

develop policies to address emerging healthcare challenges in the past, it is expected that further health reform efforts will provide measures that would be effective in combating such disease pandemics that may arise in the future.

REFERENCES

Almagambetova, N. (2011). Kazakhstan primary healthcare: where do the reforms lead us? Available at: http://www.irex.org/sites/default/files/Nailya A_STG Research Brie...

Committee on Statistics, Ministry of National Economy of the Republic Kazakhstan (2016), *Socio-economic development of the Republic of Kazakhstan*, Astana.

Katsaga, A., Kulzhanov, M., Karanikolos, M., and Rechel, B. (2012). Kazakhstan: Health system overview. *In Health systems in Transition*, Karanikolos M. and Rechel, B. (eds.), Geneva: European Observatory on Health Systems and Policies.

Kulzhanov, M., and Rechel, B. (2007). Kazakhstan: health system overview. *In Health systems in Transition*, B. Rechel (Ed.), Geneva: European Observatory on Health Systems and Policies.

Ministry of Health (2011). *Health of the Population of the Republic of Kazakhstan and Performance of Health Organizations*. Astana.

Ministry of Health. (2015). *Population Health in the Republic of Kazakhstan and Activity of Healthcare Organizations in 2014*, Kazakhstan. Astana, Ministry of Health.

Ministry of Health. (2016). *Population Health in the Republic of Kazakhstan and Activity of Healthcare Organizations in 2015*, Kazakhstan. Astana, Ministry of Health

Ministry of Health (2018). *Population Health in the Republic of Kazakhstan and Activities of Healthcare Organizations in 2017*. Kazakhstan.

Ministry of Health (2020). *Population Health in the Republic of Kazakhstan and Activities of Healthcare Organizations in 2019*. Kazakhstan.

Ministry of Health of the Republic of Kazakhstan. (2002). *Health of Population and Healthcare of Republic of Kazakhstan, 1991–2001*. Astana, Ministry of Health

Ministry of Health of the Republic of Kazakhstan. (2004). *National Program of Health Reform and Development for 2005–2010, Approved by Presidential Decree on 13 September, 2004*. Astana, Ministry of Health.

National Center for Problems of Healthy Lifestyle Development. (2016). Available at: http://www.hls.kz/

OECD. (2018). *National Health Accounts of Kazakhstan*, OECD Publishing, Paris. https://doi.org/10.1787/9789264289604-en.

Pavlovskaya, O. (2013). E-healthcare system coming to Kazakhstan. Available at: http://centralasiaonline.com/en_GB/articles/caii/features/main/2013...

President of Kazakhstan. (1997). *Kazakhstan 2030: Prosperity, Security and Welfare for all People of Kazakhstan*, Almaty, President of the Republic of Kazakhstan.

President of Kazakhstan. (1998). *The Health of the Nation*, Almaty, President of Republic of Kazakhstan.

President of Kazakhstan (2010), *State Healthcare Development Program for 2011–2015 "Salamaty Kazakhstan"*. Decree of the President of the Republic of Kazakhstan No. 1113, Almaty.

President of Kazakhstan (2020). *Kazakhstan in a New Reality: Time for Action*, Nur-Sultan.

(The) World Bank. (2004). Comments on the National Program of Health Sector Reform and Development in the Republic of Kazakhstan for 2005–2010. Washington, DC, World Bank.

(The) World Bank. (2018). *World Development Indicators*. Washington, DC. World Bank.

WHO (World Health Organization). (2011). *Evaluation of the organization and provision of primary care in Kazakhstan – a survey-based project in the regions of Almaty and Zhambyl*, World Health Organization, Geneva.

(WHO) World Health Organization. (2016). *Integrated Care Models: An Overview*. WHO Regional Office for Europe, Copenhagen.

CHAPTER 6

A Review of Public Sector Reform

The transition from traditional model of public administration to new models of public governance arose due to the inadequacies of the traditional model. The theoretical foundations of traditional public administration derive from such writers as Woodrow Wilson in the United States; the Northcote-Trevelyan Report in the United Kingdom; and the bureaucratic model of Max Weber in Germany. Traditional public administration began in the late nineteenth century, became formalized somewhere between 1900 and 1920, and lasted in most Western countries until the last quarter of the twentieth century (Uddin et al. 2020; Amagoh 2011; Belle and Ongaro 2014; Dan and Pollitt 2015).

Traditional public administration is based on a hierarchical model of bureaucracy, staffed by neutral and anonymous officials, and motivated by public interest (Hughes 2003; Habibullah et al. 2016; Anttiroiko and Valkama 2016). It is based on bureaucracy rigidity and rests on control from top to bottom. The bureaucratic system has a set of rules and regulations flowing from the public law (Panjaitan et al. 2019; Peters 2001; Lodge and Gill 2011; Kalsi and Kiran 2015).

According to Peters (2001), the principles of the traditional model have the following characteristics: an apolitical civil service; hierarchy and rules; permanence and stability; an institutional civil service; internal regulation; and quality (internally and externally to the organization). The traditional model was successful in aiding the development of modern

© The Author(s), under exclusive license to Springer Nature Singapore Pte Ltd. 2021
F. E. Amagoh, *Healthcare Policies in Kazakhstan*,
https://doi.org/10.1007/978-981-16-2370-7_6

economies, and according to Pollitt and Bouckaert (2004), it was the most efficient mode of organization possible.

The model of public governance changed around the mid-1980s to a flexible, market-based form of public management. The change encompasses the role of government in society and the relationship between the government and the governed. The traditional model is no longer relevant to the needs of a rapidly changing society. It is seen as inefficient, outmoded and old, and is being replaced with new models of public management (Bhuiyan and Amagoh 2011; Kalsi and Kiran 2015; Osborne 2006; Aiken and Bode 2009).

The failure of the traditional model was partly due to the advent of globalization, the pluralization of service provision required by citizens, and complex policy problems faced by governments. Traditional public administration did not fully encompass the significance or implications of these changes. Many public bureaucracies were seen as bloated, inefficient, and self-serving (Elahi 2009; Uddin et al. 2020; Pollitt and Bouckaert 2004; Siddiquee and Mohamed 2007), ushering in new models of reform for the public sector. This encompasses the New Public Administration (NPM) and subsequently New Public Governance (NPG). These models arose in reaction to the limitations of the old public administration in adjusting to the demands of a competitive market economy (Analoui 2009; Hansen and Lindholst 2016; Mason et al. 2019; Peters 2001).

6.1   A Closer Look at Public Sector Reform

Public sector reform (PSR) consists of processes through which the state, the private sector, non-governmental organizations, and citizens interact in order to express their interests, exercise their rights and obligations, work out their differences, and cooperate to produce public goods and services for society (Huque 2005; Brinkerhoff and Brinkerhoff 2015; Antwi and Analoui 2008; Grindle 2012). In this way, public sector reform seeks to bring a fundamental challenge to the traditional model of public administration (Bhuiyan and Amagoh 2011; Pollitt 1995; Knox 2008).

Public sector reform emerged as a key agenda within public service reform initiatives in many developed countries in the early 1980s (Anttiroiko and Valkama 2016; Dunleavy et al. 2005), with many public services in developed countries delivered mainly through competitive external service providers (Hansen and Lindholst 2016; Mason et al.

2019). In developing nations, public sector reforms were introduced in the late 1980s by international aid agencies such as the World Bank and IMF (Liou 2007; Elahi 2009). Reforms in the public sector and decentralization of administrative were set as pre-requisites and benchmarks for aid assistance (Ishii et al. 2007; Panjaitan et al. 2019; Elahi 2009; Hood 1995).

Public sector reform is thus a paradigm shift from the highly bureaucratic old public management style and covers such elements as competition; cost control (efficiency); effectiveness; and greater transparency in resource allocation. It also espouses decentralization of traditional bureaucratic institutions and performance-based management amongst others (Kalsi and Kiran 2015; UNDP 1995; Saner et al. 2008; Pollitt 1995; Mason et al. 2019).

Public sector reform is an amalgam of New Public Management and New Public Governance. New Public Management consists mostly of top-down hierarchical approach of cost-cutting and efficiency. Cost containment is a key driver in the adoption of New Public Management approaches, injecting principles of competition and private sector management into how to manage the public sector. According to Osborne (2006), the key elements of the NPM are as follows:

- An attention to lessons from private-sector management;
- Emphasis on entrepreneurial leadership within public service organizations;
- A focus on input and output control, and on performance management and audit;
- The delineation of public services to their most basic units and a focus on their cost management; and
- The growth of use of markets, competition, and contracts for resource allocation and service delivery within public services.

New Public Governance incorporates elements of equity and citizen's involvement in government decision-making (Dunleavy et al. 2005; Dan and Pollitt 2015; O'Flynn 2007). It envisions a citizen-centric bottom-up and multi-actor collaborative public management (Amagoh 2011; Hood 1995; Peters 2001).

Three reasons have been identified for the ineffectiveness of New Public Management and the emergence of New Public Governance. First, by shifting from public management to public governance, the new philosophy of public service management signifies that citizens are no longer customers or top-down receivers of public services, as articulated in New Public Management. Rather citizens are partners to the governance process and should actively participate for public functions (Aiken and Bode 2009; Greve 2007; Islam 2018).

Second, by separating finance from management, the financially competitive and market-based approach that is adopted in New Public Management from theories of finance management is not equally applicable in public services (Habibullah et al. 2016; Kalsi and Kiran 2015). Third, the job nature of the public sector is principally different from that of the private sector, and as such, adoption of private sector attitudes and theories in New Public Management for rendering public services is unsuitable (Dunleavy et al. 2005; Howe 2012; Liou 2007; Uddin et al. 2020). Performing a job in the public sector depends on multiple departments and stakeholders and a need to share authority with others, including citizens (O'Flynn 2007; Saner et al. 2008; Amagoh 2011).

Consequently, PSR tries to reformulate the quality of relationships between governments and citizens. This involves a transformation of the relationships between the public sector, private agencies, and civil society organizations in policy processes, and the delivery of public services (Bhuiyan and Amagoh 2011; Siddiquee and Mohamed 2007). It advocates a redefinition of the role of government and its relationship with other sectors alongside reforms for improving the competence of the public bureaucracy (Pollitt and Bouckaert 2004; Devlin 2010; Grindle 2012). It seeks to create and maintain an effective governmental structure and procedures to formulate and implement development policies and programs, with a focus on efficiency, cost-effectiveness, and citizen involvement (Dunleavy et al. 2005; Ranerup and Henriksen 2019). Public sector reform seeks to include process accountability with accountability in terms of outcomes (Essen 2009; Knox 2008; Chowdhury and Shil 2017). This is done by seeking areas of collaborations with the private sector and civil society organizations in other to achieve better outcomes for society.

6.2   Some Features of Public Sector Reform

As mentioned, public sector reform constitutes mechanisms government can use to be more effective in its service delivery functions through intersectoral collaborations and citizen involvement. It is a paradigm change in the governance of the public sector and can be synthesized into a focus on results of public management and their impacts on citizens' welfare. To attain these outcomes, some of the measures used are decentralization, competition, efficiency, and good governance as discussed below.

6.2.1   Decentralization

One of the theoretical underpinnings of public sector reform models is the belief that decentralization and devolution of responsibilities from the center to lower levels of government will lead to more responsiveness to citizens' needs (Hughes 2003; Aiken and Bode 2009; Dunleavy et al. 2005). Decentralization has been recognized as an essential strategic policy element in the implementation of reforms, especially in developing and transitional economies. It is the restructuring of a central administrative body into lower levels, separately managed local administrative units with delegation of authorities for enhancing decision-making processes and ensuring more effective delivery of services (Howe 2012; Analoui 2009; Greve 2002; Budd 2007). Decentralization essentially replaces highly centralized hierarchical structures with devolved administrative and management environments (Bhuiyan and Amagoh 2011; OECD 1998; Waheduzzman 2019; Antwi and Analoui 2008).

According to O'Flynn (2007), decentralization creates more disaggregated and independent administrative units within and beyond the government in order to increase local responsiveness and provide locally tailored solutions. It emphasizes transfer of the decision-making process from the center to lower levels of the public sector by transferring decision rights, responsibility, and accountability from higher authorities to lower authorities at local levels (Jones et al. 2013; Dunleavy et al. 2005; Dan and Pollitt 2015). One of the arguments for decentralization is that it enhances the efficiency and effectiveness of governance by delegating authorities to administrative units which are closer to the people. This is because local administrative bodies are closest to the population, are better informed about their needs, and know how best to respond to such demands.

It places emphasis on the fact that local population can influence decisions relating to the type, level, quality, and mix of desired services, as well as the price they are willing to pay. This ultimately leads to greater citizen engagement and satisfaction (O'Flynn 2007; Amagoh 2011; Ishii et al. 2007). The capacity of institutions and political leaders to share power and responsibilities in accordance with the principles of participation, transparency, and accountability is enhanced through this process.

Another argument for decentralization is that it enhances social cohesions. As local governments are closer to the people, participation at the local level brings together a variety of stakeholders and enhances collaboration, social cohesion, and a better understanding between citizens and government. This is because decentralization provides opportunities for policies and solutions to be tailored to suit local circumstances and problems. In addition, decentralized institutions are more flexible and can respond more quickly to the changing needs of citizens (Knox 2008; Liou 2007; World Bank 1994; Grindle 2012).

Especially in healthcare, a major reason for decentralization is the belief that it has the potential to improve the quality of health services with coverage, thereby leading to increased equity in the delivery of care. Other reasons for promoting decentralization include increasing service delivery effectiveness, efficiency of resource allocation, health worker motivation, and community participation and representation in decision making (O'Flynn 2007; Ishii et al. 2007; Devlin 2010; Hood 1995). It also helps in creating a realistic and integrated health service that accommodates local preferences, controls costs of targeted health programs to improve their implementation, and reduces inequities that results in differences in healthcare delivery to rural and urban populations (Bhuiyan and Amagoh 2011; Jones et al. 2013).

There are also arguments against the notion of excessive decentralization. Such arguments contend that when services are provided by local governments, there is the risk that it will give rise to greater inequality between regions and to political fragmentation (Panjaitan et al. 2019; Uddin et al. 2020; Habibullah et al. 2016; Lodge and Gill 2011).

The effectiveness of decentralization depends on its design and the institutional, technical, and human resources development capacity arrangements governing its strategic implementation (Antwi and Analoui 2008; World Bank 2000). The goal of decentralized governance is to identify and promote those institutional arrangements that advance legislation and policies linked to effective human development and active citizenship by bringing dividends of good governance closer to the people (Ishii et al. 2007; Uddin et al. 2020; Islam 2018).

6.2.2   Competition (Quasi-Market)

An important feature in public sector reform models is the idea of competition among public service providers. This is aimed at improving innovation, reducing costs, and has sometimes been referred to as a form of quasi-market. Such a mechanism helps to strengthen governance, usually through some combination of provider competition and user choice (Hansen and Lindholst 2016; Lodge and Gill 2011; Pedersen and Rendtorff 2010). Public sector reform considers competition as a necessary condition for efficiency, customer choice, and product/service quality (Anttiroiko and Valkama 2016; Budd 2007; Howe 2012; Patricio et al. 2020).

Here, the provision of a service is undertaken by competitive providers as in pure markets, but where the purchasers of the service are financed from resources provided by the state instead of from their own private resources (Mason et al. 2019; Amagoh 2011; Knox 2008). This is in contrast to the non-market competition which exists in traditional public administration through internal accounting, benchmarking, performance comparisons, and price competition between public administration units with the goal of reducing costs (Mosebach 2009; Padro-Lorenza and Garcia-Sanchez 2010). Quasi-market competition in public sector reform models differ from the market competition in the private-sector by utilizing instruments of tendering and contracting-out to cut costs and provide services cheaply within the publicly determined criteria (Analoui 2009; Foley 2008; Saner et al. 2008; Osborne 2006). Quasi-markets arise when governments decrease their functions as both direct funder and provider of public services.

This quasi-market model uses competition as a driver for enhancing continuous learning processes towards higher efficiency. It promotes competition between providers (public or private) and choice between several alternatives by consumers. The basic quality of the provider is ensured through an accreditation process. Users of public services are given free choice between accredited providers partly or fully financed by taxes. Thus, to the provider of the service, the user is regarded as a customer just as in a private market place. This is meant to eliminate both inefficiencies arising from bureaucratic administration and poor responsiveness to users or payers (Bode et al. 2011; Elahi 2009; Mason et al. 2019).

In addition, quasi-markets help to address the problem of allocative inefficiency which occurs when services are produced for the public at suboptimal levels because of inadequate resources used to produce the service.

State-run services are often considered to be rather poor at making efficient use of resources, hence governments would want to develop markets that reduce the fiscal burden on the state by encouraging non-state actors to organize service delivery and enhance the perception of public value. Quasi-market competition helps to reduce costs and boost efficiency through service contracts and delegation of responsibility from administrative units to public service providers as well as internal tendering for public services (Huque 2005; Bode et al. 2011; Belle and Ongaro 2014).

6.2.3   Efficiency

Increased fiscal stress faced by governments led to calls for more efficient modes of governance and public service delivery. In the public sector, there is an imbalance between the demand for public welfare services, public expenditures, and available resources (Pedersen and Rendtorff 2010; Pollitt 1995; Brinkerhoff and Brinkerhoff 2015; Devlin 2010; Howe 2012; Knox 2008). Budget constraints have increased the pressures on governments to come up with ways that would improve efficiency gains. The concern about the ineffectiveness and inefficiency in the public sector are generally associated with bureaucracy, lack of competence in some cases, and the very nature of public organizations. These concerns led to a considerable loss of confidence in the public sector with regard to its performance and generated calls for public institutions to apply principles of economy, effectiveness, and efficiency (Padro-Lorenza and Garcia-Sanchez 2010; Mosebach 2009; Lo Sorto 2013; Peters 2001). Deep budget cuts and regulatory pressures in many countries have also put pressures on the public sector to improve efficiency at all levels, with a major focus on operational functions.

It is therefore argued that by implementing public sector reform, the public sector can be more economically efficient (Hood 1995; Dunleavy et al. 2005; Greve 2008; Chowdhury and Shil 2017; Hughes 2003). Public welfare institutions should learn how to integrate value-driven management, stakeholder management, ethics, and private economic efficiency into their operations (Devlin 2010; Pedersen and Rendtorff 2010; Lodge and Gill 2011; Islam 2018; Patricio et al. 2020; Ranerup and Henriksen 2019). To do this, the public sector has to compete or collaborate with the private sector to meet the needs of citizens. This change process requires internal restructuring geared towards eliminating bureaucracy, adopting more rational processes, having greater autonomy in management, and so on (Pollitt and Bouckaert 2004; Siddiquee and Mohamed 2007; Siddiquee 2008). While efficiency through cost-cutting is a desired goal, it is cautioned that striving for unreasonable benchmark targets for efficiency may result in a deterioration of service quality.

6.2.4   Good Governance

The World Bank defines governance as the ability and capacity of a government to exercise its power to design, formulate, and implement policies with clear functions to manage its resources for economic and social development (World Bank 1994; Siddiquee and Mohamed 2007; Saner et al. 2008; Pollitt 1995). Similarly, the United Nations describes governance as the process of decision-making and other regulatory processes by which decisions are implemented (UNDP 1995; Hughes 2003; Howe 2012; Osborne 2006). Good governance has been defined in terms of accountability, efficiency, and effectiveness in public sector management. It has also been defined in terms of free flow of information (i.e. transparency) and a clear legal framework for ensuring social and economic development (i.e. justice, respect for human rights and liberties) (Habibullah et al. 2016; Lo Sorto 2013; Knox 2008; Kalsi and Kiran 2015).

Good governance is essential for long-term sustainable development. The outcomes of poor governance can be related to increased uncertainty, unpredictability, and instability of a country's political, economic, and social systems (World Bank 2000; Uddin et al. 2020; Peters 2001). Poor quality governance discourages domestic and foreign investments. For example, it increases indirectly, the cost of trade (i.e. transaction costs), thereby negatively affecting economic growth. Sustained long-term economic growth, which would be the ultimate goal of any government, cannot be achieved without a stable economic and political system.

Governance is regarded as good when it effectively allocates and manages resources to respond to collective problems and when a state efficiently provides quality public goods to its citizens. This requires the states to be assessed in terms of quality as well as quantity of public goods it provides to citizens (Kalsi and Kiran 2015; O'Flynn 2007; Siddiquee 2008). Promotion of gender equality, environmental sustainability, quality and accessible healthcare; exercise of personal freedom, tools of poverty reduction, violence-free environment, and so on are all products of good governance. These principles strengthen democratic institutions by free, fair, and frequent elections, a representative legislature, judiciary, and media independence from the state (Budd 2007; Elahi 2009; Ishii et al. 2007; Antwi and Analoui 2008; Devlin 2010).

The net result of a well-designed and implemented public sector reform policy is good governance. The World Bank (1994) and Uddin et al. (2020) identify four specific elements of good governance as: (1) accountability (officials being answerable for government behaviour), (2) participation (the involvement of citizens in the development process), (3) predictability (a legal environment that is conducive to development), and (4) transparency (readily available information to the public as well as clarification of government rules, regulations, and decisions). Similarly, Saner et al. (2008) identify four elements of governance as: the importance of networks; the change from control to influence; the blending of public and private resources; and the use of multiple instruments in developing and implementing public policies.

Consequently, it can be surmised that good governance embraces policies of economic liberalization, creation of market-friendly environments, and measures to promote and safeguard long-term global issues like education, health, and the environment (Siddiquee and Mohamed 2007; Saner et al. 2008; Patricio et al. 2020; Mosebach 2009). It is epitomized by open and enlightened policymaking, and a bureaucracy imbued with a professional and competent civil service (UNESC 2008; UNDP 1995; Smith 2010; Knox 2008; Amagoh 2011; Osborne 2007; World Bank 2000).

6.2.5   Partnerships

Partnerships vary depending on the degree of formality, permanence, private-sector involvement, and voluntariness (Aiken and Bode 2009; Greve 2007; Howe 2012). Thus, some local partnerships may be informal and voluntary, whereas others may be based on formal contracts or even legal requirements (Osborne 2007; Blair 2005; Smith 2010; Aiken and Bode 2009). Strong collaborations between the private and public sectors and civil society organizations offer ways of delivering public services faster at significant cost savings compared with conventional means (Saner et al. 2008; Siddiquee 2008). The continuous reforms of social and health service structures underline the significance of the partnership of the public and private sectors and civil society organizations (Solheim-Kile and Wald 2020; Smith 2010; Hughes 2003). Such forms of connections nurture innovation and engender new forms of service delivery that are amenable to the needs of the population. Partnerships allow inclusion of wider range of different types of co-operation arrangements between the public, private, and third sector. It is about pooling the resources of all sectors and capitalizing on the skills of the respective sectors to improve the delivery of services (Aiken and Bode 2009; Osborne 2007). Regardless of the forms they can take (e.g., social partnerships, consortia, public-private partnerships, networks), partnerships are collaborations between multiple organizations, usually from different sectors (Anttiroiko and Valkama 2016; Amagoh 2011; Siddiquee 2008).

Such inter-organizational collaboration activities are often described as responses to turbulent environments. They are organizational-level strategies to face complex, uncertain, or rapidly changing environment conditions (Mason et al. 2019; Chowdhury and Shil 2017; Budd 2007). One of the main ideas behind these partnerships is that innovation takes place where different frames and interests intersect, at the interfaces of organizations. Generally, the purpose is to build a partnership model that creates and captures value by combining and coordinating partners' heterogeneous resources (people, knowledge, finance, and technology).

Healthcare issues require new levels of strategic thinking to find innovative solutions (Solheim-Kile and Wald 2020; Anttiroiko and Valkama 2016; Hood 1995). Partnerships offer the right combination of insights and resources to address these challenges. It allows multiple sectors to share resources and bring together the diverse perspectives needed to develop solutions. Both types of organizations can benefit by combining resources and being enthusiastically innovative. By so doing, public entities must develop new approaches to meeting public health needs, and private companies must find tactics for growth and expansion that address the issues affecting their main objective, which is also greatly impacted by the rising cost of healthcare.

Governments are constantly searching for new ways to provide high-quality healthcare, but many struggle because they find it increasingly difficult to operate publicly funded healthcare facilities. Partnering with other sectors can motivate private and civil society organizations to develop new approaches that address the challenging issues facing governments in the healthcare arena.

Collaborative arrangements between government and the private sector, civil society, and other governments are therefore, one of the means to ensure that the skills and expertise needed to address societal problems are adequately harnessed for the benefit of society. PSR posits that governments must explore, assess, and engage in opportunities for collaboration both within and outside the public sector (Bhuiyan and Amagoh 2011;

Mendoza and Vernis 2008; Dan and Pollitt 2015; Lodge and Gill 2011). Governments must be prepared to work in partnerships with other public, civil society, and business organizations (Huque 2005; Ranerup and Henriksen 2019; Padro-Lorenza and Garcia-Sanchez 2010; Smith 2010). This is necessary in order to develop innovative policies that enhance cost-effective delivery of quality public services.

6.3   Conclusion

Public sector reform principles can be used to meet the healthcare needs of governments and citizens (Mosebach 2009; Lo Sorto 2013; Patricio et al. 2020) through a more people-centered and integrated care system that ensures a continuum of quality and affordable healthcare for all (WHO 2016; Belle and Ongaro 2014; Anttiroiko and Valkama 2016). Making this vision come true requires a comprehensive understanding of healthcare challenges, and a willingness to transform health systems through reforms that are based on public sector reform paradigm. The transformation of healthcare requires that governments develop policies that rethink and redesign health service systems in ways that leverage technological innovations and delivery mechanisms that are citizen-centric. This means confronting the challenges of demographic and economic constraints that may make such reforms difficult.

According to the World Bank (2016), one of the most significant concerns is an increasing elderly population. By 2030, it is estimated that 65% of the global population will be middle class (Mosebach 2009; World Bank 2016; UNDP 1995). These demographic shifts entail a change in health-related needs, with an increased prevalence of chronic diseases, mental health issues, and obesity, among others (Mosebach 2009; Howe 2012; Patricio et al. 2020; OECD 1998). Increased migration and the presence of more diverse ethnic groups in some regions can also contribute to significant stress on healthcare systems (Pedersen and Rendtorff 2010; Amagoh 2011; Waheduzzman 2019). These challenges imply that healthcare spending will continue to grow at a staggering rate. This situation has led to a push for healthcare systems to embrace a value agenda which is transparently focused on maximizing the cost-effectiveness of healthcare services (Aiken and Bode 2009; Devlin 2010; Dunleavy et al. 2005), as prescribed by public sector reform ideas. Such a change to a value-driven healthcare requires a complete overhaul of systems through policy initiatives that embrace various aspects of public sector reform.

REFERENCES

Aiken, M. and Bode, I. (2009). Killing the golden goose? third sector organizations and back-to-work programs in Germany and the UK. *Social Policy and Administration*, Vol. 18 No. 4, pp. 393–406.

Amagoh, F. (2011). New public management and healthcare reform in Kazakhstan. *International Journal of Public Administration*, Vol. 34 No. 9, pp. 567–578.

Analoui, F. (2009). Challenges of successful reform: an international perspective. *Journal of Management Development*, Vol. 28 No. 6, pp. 489–494.

Antwi, K. and Analoui, F. (2008). Challenges in building the capacity of human resource development in decentralized local governments. *Management Research News*, Vol. 31 No. 7, pp. 504–517.

Anttiroiko, A. and Valkama, P. (2016). Post-NPM-style service integration: partnership-ship based brokerage in elderly care. *International Journal of Public Sector Management*, Vol. 29 No. 7, pp. 675–689.

Belle, N. and Ongaro, E. (2014). NPM, administrative reforms and public service motivation: improving the dialogue between research agendas. *International Review of Administrative Sciences*, Vol. 80 No. 2, pp. 382–400.

Blair, H. (2005). Civil society and pro-poor initiatives in rural Bangladesh: finding a workable strategy. *World Development*, Vol. 33 No. 6, pp. 921–936

Bhuiyan, S. and Amagoh, F. (2011). Public sector reform in Kazakhstan: issues and perspectives. *International Journal of Public Sector Management*, Vol. 24 No. 3, pp. 227–249.

Bode, I., Gardin, L. and Nyssens, M. (2011). Quasi-marketization in domiciliary care: varied patterns, similar problems? *International Journal of Sociology and Social Policy*, Vol. 31 No. 3/4, pp. 222–235.

Brinkerhoff, D. and Brinkerhoff, J. (2015). Public sector management reform in developing countries: perspectives beyond NPM orthodoxy. *Public Administration and Development*, Vol. 35 No. 4, pp. 222–237.

Budd, L. (2007). Post-bureaucracy and reanimating public governance: a discourse and practice of continuity? *International Journal of Public Sector Management*, Vol. 20 No. 6, pp. 531–547.

Chowdhury, A. and Shil, N. (2017). Performance measurement systems in the context of new public management: evidence from Australian public sector and policy implications for developing countries. *Problems of Management in the 21st Century*, Vol. 12 No. 1, pp. 7–19.

Dan, S. and Pollitt, C. (2015). NPM can work: an optimistic review of the impact of new public management reforms in central and Eastern Europe. *Public Management Review*, Vol. 17 No. 9, pp. 1305–1332.

Devlin, P. (2010). Exploring efficiency's dominance: the wholeness of the process. *Quantitative Research in Accounting and Management*, Vol. 7 No. 2, pp. 141–162.

Dunleavy, P., Margetts, H., Bastow, S. and Tinkler, J. (2005). New Public Management is dead: long live digital-era governance. *Journal of Public Administration Research and Theory*, Vol. 16 No. 3, pp. 467–494.

Elahi, K. (2009). UNDP on good governance. *International Journal of Social Economics*, Vol. 36 No. 12, pp. 1167–1180.

Essen, A. (2009). New hospital payment systems: comparing medical strategies in The Netherlands, Germany and England. *Journal of Health Organizations and Management*, Vol. 23 No. 3, pp. 304–318.

Foley, J. (2008). Service delivery reform within the Canadian public sector: 1990–2002. *Employee Relations*, Vol. 3, pp. 283–303.

Greve, R. (2007). What characterize the Nordic welfare state model? *Journal of Social Sciences*, Vol. 3 No. 2, pp. 43–51.

Greve, C. (2002). New Public Management—en kort oversigt over begrebets anvendelse og udvikling. *Nordisk adminitrativt tidsskrift nr*, Vol. 88 No. 1, pp. 74–90.

Greve, C. (2008). Konkurrence—og offentlig servicelevering, FTP Dokumentation nr. 8, Kobenhavn.

Grindle, M. (2012). Public sector reform as problem-solving? Comments on the World Bank's public sector management approach for 2011–2020. *International Review of Administrative Sciences*, Vol. 79 No. 3, pp. 398–405.

Habibullah, M., Din, B., and Hamid, B. (2016). Good governance and crime rates in Malaysia. *International Journal of Social Economics*, Vol. 43 No. 3, pp. 308–320.

Hansen, M. and Lindholst, A. (2016). Marketization revisited. *International Journal of Public Sector Management*, Vol. 29 No. 5, pp. 398–408.

Hood, C. (1995). The new public management in the 1980s: variations on a theme. *Accounting, Organizations and Society*, Vol. 20 No. 2/3, pp. 93–109.

Howe, B. (2012). Governance in the interest of the most vulnerable. *Public Admin. Dev.*, Vol. 32 No. 4–5, pp. 345–356.

Hughes, O. (2003). *Public Management and Administration: An Introduction*, Palgrave Macmillan, Hampshire.

Huque, A. (2005). Explaining the myth of public sector reform in South Asia: De-linking cause and effect. *Policy and Society*, Vol. 24 No. 3, pp. 97–121.

Ishii, R., Hossain, F., & Rees, C. (2007). Participation in decentralized local governance: two contrasting case from the Philippines. *Public Organization Review*, Vol. 7, pp. 359–373.

Islam, S. (2018). New public management-based reform in Bangladesh: a review of public administration reform commission. *Indian Journal of Public Administration*, Vol. 64 No. 1, pp. 15–35

Jones, S., Aryal, K. and Collins, A. (2013). Local-level governance of risk and resilience in Nepal. *Disasters*, Vol. 37 No. 3, pp. 442–467.

Kalsi, N. and Kiran, R. (2015). "A strategic framework for good governance through e-governance optimization." *Program, Electronic Libraries, and Information Systems*, Vol. 49 No. 2, pp. 170–204.

Knox, C. (2008). Kazakhstan: Modernizing government in the context of political inertia. *International Review of Administrative Sciences*, Vol. 74 No. 3, pp. 477–496.

Liou, K. (2007). Applying good governance concept to promote local economic development: Contribution and challenges. *International Journal of Economic Development*, Vol. 9 No. 1/2, pp. 1–31.

Lodge, M. and Gill, D. (2011). Toward a new era of administrative reform? The myth of post-NPM in New Zealand. *Governance: An International Journal of Policy, Administration, and Institutions*, Vol. 24 No. 1, pp. 141–166.

Lo Sorto, C. (2013). Benchmarking operational efficiency in the integrated water service provision: does contract type matter? *Benchmarking: An International Journal*, Vol. 21 No. 6, pp. 917–943.

Mason, C., Roy, M. and Carey, G. (2019). Social enterprises in quasi-markets: exploring the critical gap. *Social Enterprise Journal*, Vol. 15 No. 3, pp. 358–375.

Mendoza, X., and Vernis, A. (2008), The changing role of governents and the emergence of the relational state. *Corporate Governance*, Vol. 8 No. 4, pp. 389–396.

Mosebach, K. (2009), "Commercializing German hospital care: effects of new public management and managed care under neoliberal conditions", *German Policy Studies*, Vol. 5 No. 1, pp. 65–98.

OECD. (1998). *Public Management Reform and Economic and Social Development.* PUMA, Paris: OECD.

O'Flynn, J. (2007). From new public management to public value: paradigmatic change and managerial implications. *Australian Journal of Public Administration*, Vol. 66 No. 3, pp. 353–366.

Osborne, S. (2006). The new public governance. *Public Management Review*, Vol. 8 No. 3, pp. 377–387.

Osborne, S. (2007). *Public-Private Partnerships: Theory and Practice in International Perspective*, Routledge, London.

Padro-Lorenza, J. and Garcia-Sanchez, I. (2010). Effect of operation size, environmental conditions and management on municipal sewerage services. *International Journal of Productivity and Performance Management*, Vol. 59 No. 3, pp. 206–228.

Panjaitan, R., Sarwono, S., and Saleh, C. (2019). The role of central government and local government and the moderating effect of good governance on forest fire policy in Indonesia. *Benchmarking: An International Journal*, Vol. 26 No. 1, pp. 147–159.

Patricio, L., Sangiorgi, D., Mahr, D., Carc, M., Kalantari, S. and Sundar, S. (2020). Leveraging service design for healthcare transformation: toward people-centered integrated, and technology-enabled healthcare systems. *Journal of Service Management*, Vol. 31 No. 5, pp. 889–909.

Pedersen, J. and Rendtorff, J. (2010). Balancing values and economic efficiency in the public sector: what can public welfare service institutions learn from private service firms? *Social and Business Review*, Vol. 5 No. 3, pp. 293–302.

Peters, B. (2001). *The Future of Governing*. University Press of Kansas, Lawrence, Kansas.

Pollitt, C. (1995). Justification by works or by faith: evaluating the New Public Management. *Evaluation*, Vol. 1 No. 2, pp. 133–154.

Pollitt, C. and Bouckaert, G. (2004). *Public Management Reform: A Comparative Analysis*, Oxford: Oxford University Press.

Ranerup, A. and Henriksen, H. (2019). Enrolling citizens as informed consumers in quasi-markets. *Information Technology & People*, Vol. 32 No. 6, pp. 1517–1535.

Saner, R., Toseva, G., Atamanov, A., & Sahov, A. (2008). Government governance (GG) and inter-ministerial policy coordination (IMPC) in Eastern and Central Europe and Central Asia. *Public Organization Review: A Global Journal*, Vol. 8 No. 3, pp. 215–231.

Siddiquee, N., and Mohamed, M. (2007). Paradox of public sector reforms in Malaysia: a good governance perspective. *Public Administration Quarterly*, Vol. 31 No. 3, pp. 284–313.

Siddiquee, N. (2008). Service delivery innovations and governance: the Malaysian experience. *Transforming Government: People, Process and Policy*, Vol. 2 No. 3, pp. 194–213.

Smith, S. (2010). Hybridization and non-profit organizations: the governance challenge. *Policy and Society*, Vol. 29 No. 3, pp. 219–229.

Solheim-Kile, E. and Wald, Andreas (2020). Public-private joint ventures in the healthcare sector: enlarging the shadow of the future through social and economic incentives. *International Journal of Public Sector Management*, (online first version). https://doi.org/10.1108/IJPS-12-20190318.

Uddin, M., Haque, C., and Khan, M. (2020). Good governance and local level policy implementation for disaster-risk-reduction: actual, perpetual and contested perspectives in coastal communities in Bangladesh. *Disaster Prevention and Management: An International Journal*, (online first version). https://doi.org/10.1108/DPM-03-2020-0069.

UNDP (United Nations Development Program). (1995). Public Sector Management, Governance and Sustainable Human Development, World Bank: Washington, DC.

UNESC (United Nations Economic and Social Council) (2008). National Report on the Achievement of Kazakhstan's Strategic Priorities to 2030 in the light of the Millennium Development Goals. Available at: www.apps01.un.org/nvpcms.

Waheduzzman, W. (2019). Challenges in transitioning from new public management to new public governance in a developing country context. *International Journal of Public Sector Management*, Vol. 32 No. 7, pp. 689–705.

(The) World Bank. (1994). Governance: The World Bank's Experience, Washington, DC, World Bank.

(The) World Bank. (2000). Reforming public institutions and strengthening governance: A World Bank strategy. Washington, DC, World Bank.

World Bank (2016). *WDI -World Development Indicators*. Available at: http://data.worldbank.org/products/wdi.

WHO (World Health Organization). (2016). *Integrated Care Models: An Overview*. WHO Regional Office for Europe, Copenhagen.

CHAPTER 7

Features of Public Sector Reform in Kazakhstan's Health Reform Programs

Several aspects of public sector reform are evident in Kazakhstan's health reform programs. As mentioned earlier in the previous chapter, public sector reform gained prominence in the West in the 1980s, and was not part of the governance model of the Soviet Union. This chapter examines elements of public sector reform that can be deduced from the various reform programs in Kazakhstan's health system. It focuses on the following: decentralization and devolution of health delivery responsibilities; efficiency; quality; education and training of health professionals; and competition.

7.1 Decentralization and Devolution of Responsibilities

One of the primary aims of public sector reform principles in post-Soviet Kazakhstan is the move from hierarchical and centralized service delivery system to arrangements where services are delivered in ways that are more responsive to citizens' needs (Birtanov 2016; Analoui 2009). Decentralization has been shown to constitute one of the strategic policy elements in the implementation of health reforms in developing and transitional economies (Amagoh 2011; Hughes 2003; Ishii et al. 2007; Witesman and Wise 2009). Since Kazakhstan's independence, its healthcare system has undergone various forms of decentralization, although the

F. E. Amagoh, *Healthcare Policies in Kazakhstan*, https://doi.org/10.1007/978-981-16-2370-7_7

central government has retained considerable authority. This has been mostly achieved through the privatization of some health facilities and the devolution of administrative and financial responsibilities from national level to *oblast* and sometimes *rayon* levels (Ministry of Health of the Republic of Kazakhstan 2004; Makhmutova 2001; Wilson et al. 2002). For example, The *Concept of Healthcare Reform* of 1992 states that health administration should be decentralized to regional and local levels in order to ensure that the health needs of the population are effectively addressed.

Decentralization and devolution of responsibilities was also established in the 1995 *Law on Local Self-government*, which delegates health management and financing functions to the *oblast* level (Makhmutova 2001; Kulzhanov and Rechel 2007; Perlman and Gleason 2007). The President's 1997 *Strategy Kazakhstan 2030* also empowered oblasts and local communities to develop strategies that promote healthy lifestyles and various forms of health promotion and disease prevention (President of Kazakhstan 1997). This was further emphasized by the government's establishment of the *National Center for Healthy Lifestyle* and the *Law on the Health of the Nation* in 1998. These measures were aimed at encouraging local communities to develop and promote various aspects of healthy living among the Kazakh population (Brinkerhoff 2002; President of Kazakhstan 1998; Ministry of Health of the Republic of Kazakhstan 2002).

In line with the concept of decentralization, the *National Program of Healthcare Reform and Development* which was implemented in phases from 2005 to 2010 delineated the functions between the central and regional units. It gave *oblast* authorities the responsibilities of implementing healthcare planning and operations based on policies established at the national level. As described in Chap. 4, *oblast* responsibilities include:

- Planning and allocation of resources for healthcare delivery to the population in the context of the guaranteed benefits package;
- Payment of healthcare providers;
- Delivery of general health services;
- Licensing of selected medical and pharmaceutical activities;
- centralized procurement of certain pharmaceuticals at the local level (excluding for example vaccines and immune-biological pharmaceuticals); and
- Budget formation and provider payment operations. (Ministry of Health of the Republic of Kazakhstan 2004; Kulzhanov and Rechel 2007).

On the other hand, responsibilities of the Ministry of Health, which represents the central authority include:

- Ensuring a unified national health policy;
- Performing executive functions, such as ensuring equal access to healthcare in all areas of the country to the basic benefits package;
- Setting standards for the provision of health services;
- Planning health sector development; and
- Developing the legal framework of the health system. (Ministry of Health of the Republic of Kazakhstan 2004; Kulzhanov and Rechel 2007).

Subsequent reforms also promote the decentralization of health functions. The *State Healthcare Development Program* (*Salamaty*) program implemented from 2011 to 2015 states that the effectiveness of the health sector can be enhanced by decentralizing the responsibilities of quality health provision to *oblasts'* and *rayons'* authorities and providing them with the necessary resources. In addition, the *State Policy for Public Health* (*Densaulyk*) implemented from 2016 to 2019 provides that prevention and monitoring of chronic diseases (such as cardiovascular, cancer, tuberculosis, etc.) are better managed and coordinated at regional and local levels (OECD 2018a; WHO 2015; Ministry of Health of the Republic of Kazakhstan 2015a). Finally, the *State Program for Healthcare Development* to be implemented from 2020 to 2025 emphasizes the renewal of healthcare infrastructure of the various regions with significant inputs from the regional authorities. It also provides that regional and local authorities continue to play a significant role in promoting healthy lifestyle among the population. These shifts of resources and responsibilities to regional and local administrative units have allowed local health officials to be more responsive to the healthcare needs of their jurisdictions (Prime Minister of Kazakhstan 2019; Chan et al. 2020).

7.2   EFFICIENCY

Measures to improve efficiency and quality of the health system are evident in the health reform programs. As part of the measures to improve efficiency in the health system, the *National Program for Healthcare Reform and Development 2005–2010* provides measures to reduce redundancies in the system. One of the major areas that helped to reduce costs and improve efficiency was the move from inpatient to outpatient care. The reliance on inpatient care as inherited from the Soviet era led to significant excess capacity in the hospital sector and substantial wastes in resources. The outpatient provider system emphasized in the health reform was significant in reducing wastes of resources and duplication of services and led to significant savings in the health system (Aringazina et al. 2012; Committee on Statistics, Ministry of National Economy of the Republic of Kazakhstan 2016; Ministry of Health of the Republic of Kazakhstan 2016). The reform further improved efficiency by promoting a patient-centered family medicine approach in primary healthcare and improving disease prevention methods. Other efficiency measures in the *National Program for Healthcare Reform and Development 2005–2010* include: an improved compensation system for healthcare workers based on performance; an enhanced framework for reimbursing providers of the state-guaranteed benefits package; and standardization of health services by including evidence-based diagnosis and treatment protocols (Ministry of Health of the Republic of Kazakhstan 2004).

The *State Healthcare Development Program for 2011–2015 (Salamaty)* also placed much emphasis on the efficiency of the health system by facilitating improvements in technical aspects of health facilities, and specifying what constitutes guaranteed benefits package for inpatient care. This reform also focused on improving the development of telemedicine and the use of aviation to improve health services in remote and inaccessible areas of the country (Danilovich and Yessaliyeva 2014; Ministry of Health of the Republic of Kazakhstan 2015; www.pmb.kz).

The goal of efficiency and quality was also stated in the *State Policy for Public Health (Densaulyk)*, which was implemented from 2016 to 2019. The *State Policy for Public Health* aimed to efficiently strengthen the health system in ways that would ensure socioeconomic development (OECD 2018; Ministry of Health of the Republic of Kazakhstan 2015: Danilovich and Yessaliyeva 2014). This was to be achieved by improving prevention and control mechanisms for preventable diseases. The reform emphasized the importance of healthy lifestyles and creation of centers of best practices for primary healthcare around the country.

Kazakhstan's most recent health reform program, the *State Program for Healthcare Development 2020–2025* has measures to improve efficiency by reducing redundancies and improving the quality of healthcare delivered to citizens in a cost-effective manner. This reform introduced a mandatory health insurance for all citizens effective January 1, 2020, to ensure basic health coverage for the population. It encourages preventive health measures through regular medical checkups in order to forestall illnesses that would be costlier for individuals and the government in the long-run (Prime Minister of Kazakhstan 2019).

7.3   QUALITY

With regard to quality improvements in Kazakhstan's healthcare system, the various healthcare reforms have made significant efforts in improving the quality of healthcare delivery in Kazakhstan. Perhaps the healthcare reform that took a more comprehensive approach to improve the quality of healthcare in Kazakhstan is the *National Program for Healthcare Reform and Development 2005–2010*. In line with quality initiatives in public sector reform, the reform established several quality indicators, such as the UK's comprehensive performance assessment (CPA) framework aimed at reporting on the quality of public services performance data in all areas of the public sector, including healthcare (Knox 2008; Amagoh 2011; Aringazina et al. 2012).

The focus on improving service quality in the public sector, particularly in healthcare, was emphasized in a Presidential decree in 2007 titled: *Measures aimed at Modernizing Public Administration System in the Republic of Kazakhstan*. The measures in the decree include improving the quality of processes, procedures, and public service provision and improving the professional skills, efficiency, and coordination of all state apparatuses (Ismailova et al. 2010; Amagoh 2011). A new drug formulary system was introduced in 2009 to enhance the procurement of pharmaceuticals with a focus on evidence-based medicine, quality, safety, and effectiveness (Rechel et al. 2012; Kumar et al. 2013; IMF 2014).

Based on the provisions of the *National Program for Healthcare Reform and Development 2005–2010*, a rigorous accreditation process was introduced in 2009 which enabled Kazakhstan to become a member of the *International Society for Quality in Health Care (ISQUA)*. This provision required public and private service providers, including hospitals, to undergo a formal process of quality accreditation in order to be part of the national healthcare system, and be qualified to receive public funding within the State Guaranteed Benefits Package (Birtanov 2016; Danilovich and Yessaliyeva 2014; IMF 2014). For medical practitioners and specialists, a parallel process of reaccreditation was introduced in 2012, with a requirement for renewal every five years (Ministry of Health of the Republic of Kazakhstan 2015).

The *State Healthcare Development Program for 2011–2015 (Salamaty)* emphasizes the importance of quality in the health system by giving the Ministry of Health the responsibility for:

- Developing national policies on quality assurance and accreditation for healthcare facilities;
- Developing the legislative basis for the accreditation of health organizations;
- Developing measures for quality control of health services and efficiency of all health organizations;
- Introducing a quality management system at all levels of healthcare;
- Developing a system of licensing and accreditation of health facilities;
- Providing a differentiated payment system that takes account of the quality of services provided; and
- Publishing ratings of healthcare providers in the mass media. (Katsaga et al. 2012; www.pmb.kz)

Under this reform, the *Committee for Health Services Quality Control* was established at the national level to consider citizens' complaints on quality of health services provided (Pavlovskaya 2013; Committee on Statistics, Ministry of National Economy of the Republic of Kazakhstan 2016; Kumar et al. 2013).

7.4   EDUCATION AND TRAINING OF HEALTH PROFESSIONALS

The goals of public sector reform cannot be achieved without a skilled, well-educated and professional workforce. The health reform programs are aimed to continuously improve the training and skills of health workers and the coordination of health delivery functions (Ministry of Health of the Republic of Kazakhstan 2004; Knox 2008; World Bank 2010).

The process of modernizing the skills and competence of the workforce in the health sector began with *The Concept of Healthcare Reform* of 1992 which emphasized the importance of improved training of healthcare professionals. In line with the emphasis on education and training of health professionals, the *Law on the Health System* in 2003 gave the Ministry of Health the responsibility of approving forms and training programs for medical specialties and defining standards for the training of specialists with higher and postgraduate education, amongst others (Ministry of Health of the Republic of Kazakhstan 2004; Kulzhanov and Rechel 2007: Kumar et al. 2013).

This was followed by the *National Program for Healthcare Reform and Development 2005–2010* which aimed to improve the quality and training of health professionals by bringing it up to international standards. Based on this reform, the *Concept for the Reform of Medical and Pharmaceutical Training for 2006–2010* was issued in 2007 to provide new standards for the training of medical and pharmacy students. This also provided for more robust training of hospital administrators and health managers in order to improve the administrative competence of the managerial staff of healthcare facilities (Knox 2008; OECD 2016; World Bank 2004).

The *State Healthcare Development Program for 2011–2015 (Salamaty)* also established procedures and standards for accreditation of basic medical education in line with international best practices. For example, it ensured that health education in Kazakhstan met the standards of *World Federation of Medical Education (WFME)*. This led to the inclusion of several public medical educational institutions in Kazakhstan to be included in the *World Health Organization's World Directory of Medical Schools* (Ministry of Health of the Republic of Kazakhstan 2015; World Bank 2016; www.pmb.kz).

The *State Health Development Program 2016–2019 (Densaulyk)* emphasized the modernization of medical education by updating state standards at all levels of medical and pharmaceutical education based on international best practices and full digitalization of medical educational facilities. It also established the *Competence Model for Teachers of Medical and Pharmaceutical institutions of Higher Education* to improve the skills and competence of the workforce in the health sector. Furthermore, the reform facilitated strategic partnerships of medical universities in Kazakhstan with leading foreign medical educational institutions, such as the strategic partnership of Astana Medical University with La Sapienza Rome University, one of the largest and best universities in Europe and the world (IMF 2017; www.amu.kz).

Finally, the *State Program of Development of Healthcare of the Republic of Kazakhstan 2020–2025* aims to promote strategic partnerships and faculty exchanges (academic mobility) with foreign medical universities in order to expose the Kazakhstan's medical professionals to the best practices and medical working conditions in Western countries (Prime Minister of Kazakhstan 2019). Table 7.1 shows the number of physicians and nurses in Kazakhstan from 1990 to 2015. As can be seen from Table 7.1, the number of physicians and nurses and midwives (per 1000 population) as well as the number of dentists (per 10,000 population) decreased from 1990 to 2015. While this decrease is evident, it is compensated by the increase in the quality of healthcare that is been provided compared to the Soviet era. This is because of significant investments that Kazakhstan has made in advanced medical technologies and innovations in the healthcare delivery system. There is also a significant increase in the professionalism and competence of healthcare professionals and the impacts of Western best practices in healthcare provision brought about by the healthcare reform programs. That said, Kazakhstan is making efforts to increase the number of healthcare professionals to a level that would meet the healthcare needs of the population.

7.5   COMPETITION

Public sector reform requires a competitive environment in the provision of public services as a necessary condition for quality, efficiency, and effectiveness. Competition is regarded as one of the cornerstones of good governance. While the idea of a competitive environment was absent during the Soviet years, the government of Kazakhstan has made efforts to create a competitive environment in its healthcare system (Aringazina et al. 2012; Kulzhanov and Rechel 2007; World Bank 2004). Such measures include the introduction of patient choice of hospitals and doctors; increased

Table 7.1 Number of selected healthcare professionals in Kazakhstan, 1990–2015 (selected years)

	1990	1995	2000	2005	2010	2011	2012	2013	2014	2015
Physicians (per 1000 population)	4.05	3.80	3.28	3.61	3.93	3.95	3.91	3.95	3.98	–
Nurses and midwives (per 1000 population)	10.05	9.44	6.17	6.88	7.72	7.92	8.06	8.03	7.2	7.29
Dentists (per 10,000 population)	4.23	4.24	2.65	3.39	4.09	3.96	4.13	3.76	3.71	2.89

Source: World Bank (www.worldbank.org); Katsaga et al. (2012); Kulzhanov and Rechel (2007)

financial autonomy of public healthcare providers; encouraging private sector practice; ensuring that state-owned and private healthcare providers have the same entitlements when providing the State-Guaranteed Basic Benefits Package; and facilitating the transition of some public providers to government enterprises and joint-stock companies (Ministry of Health of the Republic of Kazakhstan 2004; Amagoh 2011; OECD 2018a). State enterprises can charge fees for certain services and have financial autonomy as opposed to state facilities which are wholly financed by the state budget. These measures have created a competitive environment in the healthcare system by encouraging medical institutions and practitioners to be innovative and efficient in their service delivery. This competition has led to better service delivery among healthcare providers in their quest to attract more customers.

7.6   Conclusion

The drive to achieve a modernized healthcare system that meets the needs of its citizens facilitated Kazakhstan's efforts for continuous health reform policies. Each of the reforms is targeted at parts of the health system in need of improved efficiency and effectiveness. In trying to meet the healthcare needs of the population, the reforms are derived from public sector reform paradigm which consists of decentralization; efficiency; quality; education and training of healthcare professionals; and competition.

The reforms have significantly improved the health system of Kazakhstan. Decentralization of health delivery responsibilities has ensured that local and regional authorities are in a position to quickly and effectively respond to the healthcare needs of the population (of course, with direction from the central government). The efficiency and quality provisions in the reforms facilitate cost-effectiveness in the health delivery system without compromising quality of healthcare products and services. Education and training of health professionals has brought in western best practices in the health educational institutions in the country and improved the competence and professionalism of healthcare workers in line with international standards. Similarly, the provision in the health reforms that encourages competition in the health system has given citizens the ability to choose more innovative providers that would meet their healthcare needs at reasonable costs.

REFERENCES

Amagoh, F. (2011). New public management and healthcare reform in Kazakhstan. *International Journal of Public Administration*, Vol. 34 No. 9, pp. 567–578.

amu.kz. Implementation of the state health development program *"densaulyk"* for 2016–2019. (available at: www.amu.kz/en/program-densaulyk-implementation.php).

Analoui, F. (2009). Challenges of successful reform: an international perspective. *Journal of Management Development*, Vol. 28 No. 6, pp. 489–494.

Aringazina, A., Gulis, G., and Allegrante, J. (2012). Public health challenges and priorities for Kazakhstan. *Central Asian Journal of Global Health*, Vol. 1 No. 1 (available at: http://cajgh.pitt.edu).

Birtanov Y. (2016). Kazakhstan gears up to launch social health insurance. *Bulletin of the World Health Organization*, Vol. 94, pp. 792–793, https://doi.org/10.2471/BLT.16.031116.

Brinkerhoff, D. (2002). Government-nonprofit partners for health sector reform in Central Asia: family group practitioners in Kazakhstan and Kyrgyzstan. *Public Administration and Development*, Vol. 22 No. 1, pp. 51–61.

Chan, B., Rausher, C., Issina, A., Kozhageldiyeva, L., Kuzembaeva, D., Davies, C., Kravchenko, H., Hindmarsh, M., McGowan, J., and Kulkaeva, G. (2020). "A program to improve quality of care for patients with chronic diseases, Kazakhstan", *Bulletin of the World Health Organization*, Vol. 98, pp. 161–169.

Committee on Statistics, Ministry of National Economy of the Republic of Kazakhstan (2016), *Socio-economic development of the Republic of Kazakhstan*, Astana.

Danilovich, N. and Yessaliyeva, E. (2014). Effects of out-of-pocket payments on access to maternal health services in Almaty, Kazakhstan: a qualitative study. *Europe-Asia Studies*, Vol. 66, pp. 578–589.

Hughes, O. (2003). *Public Management and Administration: An Introduction*, Palgrave Macmillan, Hampshire.

IMF. (2014). *Republic of Kazakhstan, Selected Issues*, IMF Country Report No. 14/243.

IMF. (2017). *World Economic Outlook Databases*. International Monetary Fund.

Ishii, R., Hossain, F., and Rees, C. (2007). Participation in decentralized local governance: two contrasting case from the Philippines. *Public Organization Review*, Vol. 7, pp. 359–373.

Ismailova, G., Aydarhanova, K., Demessinov, A. and Aubakirova, A. (2010). Health economic rates for medical services and clinical economic analysis as components of health reform in Kazakhstan. *Medical and Health Sciences Journal*, Vol. 1, pp. 1–7.

Katsaga, A., Kulzhanov, M., Karanikolos, M., and Rechel, B. (2012). Kazakhstan: Health system overview. *In Health systems in Transition*, Karanikolos M. and

Rechel, B. (eds.), Geneva: European Observatory on Health Systems and Policies.

Knox, C. (2008). Kazakhstan: modernizing government in the context of political inertia. *International Review of Administrative Sciences,* Vol. 74 No. 3, pp. 477–496.

Kulzhanov, M., and Rechel, B. (2007). Kazakhstan: health system overview. *In Health systems in Transition,* B. Rechel (Ed.), Geneva: European Observatory on Health Systems and Policies.

Kumar, A., Izekenova, and Abikulova, A. (2013). "Inpatient care in Kazakhstan: A comparative analysis" *J Res Med Sci.* Vol. 18, No. 7, pp. 549–553, (available at: http://www.ncbi.nlm.nih.gov/pmc/articles/PMC3897019).

Makhmutova, M. (2001). Local government in Kazakhstan. In Munteanu, I. and Popa, V. (Eds.) *Developing New Rules in Old Environment: Local Government in Eastern Europe, in the Caucasus and in the Central Asia,* The Open Society, Budapest, Chapter 8, pp. 431–447.

Ministry of Health of the Republic of Kazakhstan. (2015). *Population Health in the Republic of Kazakhstan and Activity of Health Care Organizations in 2014,* Kazakhstan.

Ministry of Health of the Republic of Kazakhstan. (2015a). *National Health Accounts of the Republic of Kazakhstan, a Report on Healthcare Expenditure for the Year 2014,* Kazakhstan.

Ministry of Health of the Republic of Kazakhstan. (2016), *Population Health in the Republic of Kazakhstan and Activity of Health Care Organizations in 2015,* Kazakhstan.

Ministry of Health of the Republic of Kazakhstan. (2002), *Health of Population and Health care of Republic of Kazakhstan, 1991–2001.* Astana, Ministry of Health.

Ministry of Health of the Republic of Kazakhstan. (2004), *National Program of Health Reform and Development for 2005–2010, Approved by Presidential Decree on 13 September, 2004.* Kazakhstan.

OECD (2018), *National Health Accounts of Kazakhstan,* OECD Publishing, Paris.

OECD (2018a), *OECD Reviews of Health Systems: Kazakhstan.* OECD Publishing, Paris

OECD (2016), *Multi-dimensional Review of Kazakhstan: Volume 1. Initial Assessment,* OECD Publishing, Paris,

pm.kz. Salamaty, national healthcare development program. (available at: http://www.pm.kz/program/about/index/7&lang=en).

Pavlovskaya, O. (2013). E-healthcare system coming to Kazakhstan. (available at: http://centralasiaonline.com/en_GB/articles/caii/features/main/2013...).

Perlman, B., & Gleason, G. (2007). Cultural determinism versus administrative logic: Asian values and administrative reform in Kazakhstan and Uzbekistan. *Intl Journal of Public Administration,* 30, 1–16.

President of Kazakhstan. (1997). *Kazakhstan 2030: Prosperity, Security and Welfare for all People of Kazakhstan,* Almaty, President of the Republic of Kazakhstan.

President of Kazakhstan. (1998). *The Health of the Nation,* Almaty, President of Republic of Kazakhstan.

Prime Minister of Kazakhstan. (2019). *Emphasis on Healthy Lifestyles and Human Capital: About the Program of Healthcare Development 2020–2025.* Nur-Sultan, Kazakhstan.

Rechel, B., Ahmedov, M., Akkazieva, B., Katsaga, A., Khojamurodov, G. and McKee, M. (2012). Lessons from Two Decades of Health Reform in Central Asia", *Health Policy and Planning,* Vol. 27, pp. 281–287.

Wilson, J., Gardner, D., Kurganbaeva, G., and Sakharchuk, E. (2002). The changing role of local government managers in a transitional economy: evidence from the Republic of Kazakhstan. *The International Journal of Public Sector Management,* Vol. 15 No. 5, pp. 399–441.

Witesman, E. and Wise, C. (2009). The centralization/decentralization paradox in civil service reform: how government structure affects democratic training of civil servants. *Public Administration Review,* Vol. 69 No. 1, pp. 116–127.

(The) World Bank. (2004). *Comments on the National Program of Health Sector Reform and Development in the Republic of Kazakhstan for 2005–2010.* Washington, DC, World Bank.

(The) World Bank. (2010). *Kazakhstan: Data and Statistics.* (available at: www.worldbank.org.kz/website/external/countries/ecaext/kazakhstan).

(The) World Bank. (2016). *WDI-World Development indicators.* (available at: http://data.worldbank.org/products/wdi).

WHO (World Health Organization). (2015). *Ambulatory Care Sensitive Conditions in Kazakhstan.* World Health Organization, Geneva.

CHAPTER 8

Partnerships and Collaborations

Kazakhstan, like many governments around the world, is finding ways to partner with the private and nonprofit sectors as well as international organizations in developing an efficient and effective healthcare delivery system (Ovcharenko 2004; Nafissa 2020; Ministry of Health of the Republic of Kazakhstan 2002; President of Kazakhstan 1997). Kazakhstan's healthcare reforms encourage collaborations between the government, civil society groups, the private sector, and international organizations. As one of the hallmarks of public sector reform, collaborations with other sector offer opportunities for governments to harness the capabilities of other sectors, as well as citizens in meeting the challenges of governance (Amagoh 2011; GerstIberger and Schneider 2013; President of Kazakhstan 1998). This chapter discusses the collaborative arrangements Kazakhstan has pursued as part of the public sector reform programs in modernizing its health system. It discusses partnerships with the private sector (in form of public–private partnerships), non-governmental organizations (NGOs), and international organizations.

8.1 NONPROFIT ORGANIZATIONS

Non-governmental organizations, in the form of civil society organizations, serve as intermediaries between the community and the state in ensuring that governments are better informed in meeting the needs of the community. Consequently, community engagement for improved

F. E. Amagoh, *Healthcare Policies in Kazakhstan*,
https://doi.org/10.1007/978-981-16-2370-7_8

service to individuals is an important dimension of integrated service delivery, which is in turn a key component of new public governance (Kabdiyeva and Dixon 2014; Civil Alliance of Kazakhstan 2011). The World Bank (2007) recognizes the potential of NGOs and the civil society organizations in the following functions:

- Ensuring that voices of the poor and marginalized are heard by governments and that their views are factored into policy decisions;
- Promoting public sector accountability and transparency;
- Developing shared visions of national development and poverty reduction strategies;
- Ensuring the provision of technical expertise and innovative and cost-efficient solutions to service delivery; and
- Delivering social services in post-conflict/post-disaster settings.

In Kazakhstan, NGOs' engagement in the health sector is multi-faceted and involves liaising between the public and the Ministry of Health. Beginning from its independence, Kazakhstan endorsed the functions of civil society as essential tools for ensuring the quality delivery of public services. As a result, citizens' involvement in public organizations were legalized in 1991, and, in 2001, a law was passed allowing not-for-profit organizations to pursue civil undertakings (Makhmutova and Akhmetova 2011; Ovcharenko 2004).

Moreover, Kazakhstan has adopted a number of legislations and ratified many international conventions, which encourage the growth of civil society; some of them are: the ratification in 2001 of the Optional Protocol to the UN convention on "Child Rights" and on "Married Women's Citizenship"; and six ILO conventions among which are: Equal Remuneration Convention; Minimum Age Convention, and Abolition of forced Labor Convention (Alymkulova and Seipulnick 2005; Kabdiyeva and Dixon 2014).

The 1994 Law on Trade Unions allowed the freedom to register and form trade unions. This includes the *Health Workers Union* which is considered as one of the largest unions in the country. The *Health Workers Union* works closely with the government and is consulted on health policy issues (Kazakhstan 2006).

NGOs in the health sector focus mostly on health-promotion activities and patients with chronic diseases or people in high-risk groups. Some NGOs in Kazakhstan were awarded grants from the *Global Fund* to fight diseases such as AIDS, Tuberculosis, Malaria, and so on. In 2005, the government passed the *Social Procurement Arrangements Act* which created a legal basis for effective partnership between the state and civil society (Diachenko 2008; Amagoh 2011). NGOs contribute significantly to the development of health policies, legislation, and regulation, and were significant in contributing to the establishment of the *Code on People's Health and the Healthcare System*. The Kazakhstan *Medical Pedagogical Association* helps in the development and implementation of state programs aimed at improving child and maternal health, reproductive health, and health promotion (Brinkerhoff 2002; Ovcharenko 2004).

According to provisions of the *National Program of Health Care Reform and Development for 2005–2010*, the Ministry of Health is empowered to involve NGO representatives in the process of professional revalidation of health workers and the independent quality control of healthcare (Ministry of Health of the Republic of Kazakhstan 2004; Amagoh 2011; Buxton 2009). Such collaborations incorporate features, such as performance standards for service delivery, sharing of staff between public sector agencies and NGOs, innovations intended to increase incentives for service providers, and the participation of NGOs in health sector policymaking. For example, in 2005 the Government for the first time started to allocate public funds to NGOs working predominantly on the prevention of "socially significant" conditions, the rehabilitation of patients, and the prevention of drug use (Kulzhanov and Rechel 2007; Katsaga et al. 2012). Some of the most active NGOs in the health sector in Kazakhstan include:

- Diabetes Association of the Republic of Kazakhstan;
- Kazakhstan Association of Family Physicians;
- National Association of Nurses;
- Dara Foundation, which focuses on children with disabilities and assists with children health facilities;
- Ayala Charity Foundation, which helps with children's health and educations;
- Aman-Saulyk, which focuses on health and social protection for the population;
- Akinyet Fund helps children with disabilities; and
- Family Group Practitioners Association (FGPA), which is another important NGO group in the health sector.

Devolution of some regulatory functions and shared interests in innovative approaches to quality control and monitoring established in the health reforms gave FGPAs significant roles in establishing quality-of-care standards, monitoring performance, and accreditation of healthcare providers. This has made a significant difference in the speed and effectiveness of primary healthcare services reform in Kazakhstan (Kulzhanov and Rechel 2007; Makhmutova and Akhmetova 2011).

8.2   International Organizations

Since its independence, international organizations and donor agencies have played a vital role in modernizing Kazakhstan's healthcare system. Cooperation with international organizations is one of the key development strategies of Kazakhstan's health sector (Bergamaschi et al. 2017; Adams and Garbutt 2008). These collaborative arrangements have allowed Kazakhstan to develop its healthcare infrastructure in addition to making efforts to meet global standards and western best practices.

The *National Program of Health Care Reform and Development for 2005–2010* made provisions to improve coordination of funds, shared expertise, and other development assistance from international donor agencies. It empowered the Ministry of Health to collaborate with a number of international donor agencies, such as The World Bank; World Health Organization (WHO); the United States Agency for International Development (USAID); United Nations International Children Emergency Fund (UNICEF); United Nations Development Program (UNDP); the United Nations Population Fund (UNFPA); the European Union; United Kingdom Department for International Development (DFID); and so on (Ministry of Health of the Republic of Kazakhstan 2004).

Major projects have been undertaken by these donor agencies in the areas of primary care, health financing and new provider payment systems, priority programs on issues such as family planning, safe motherhood, TB, HIV/AIDS, disease prevention and health promotion campaigns and so on, and these have led to significant improvements in health indicators in Kazakhstan (Ministry of National Economy of the Republic of Kazakhstan: Statistics Committee 2018; Abdymanapov et al. 2016).

The World Bank continuously provides technical assistance to the Ministry of Health in determining strategic priorities of health reform and for the improvement of the health management system. For example, in 2009 the World Bank instituted the *Health Sector Technology Transfer and*

Institutional Reform project in Kazakhstan at a cost of $296 million. The project brought international best practices in healthcare to Kazakhstan by building up the capacity of specialists in health financing, healthcare quality, information systems, and public health (World Bank 2012).

In 2009, the Ministry of Health signed a Memorandum of Understanding on healthcare cooperation with the US Agency for International Development (USAID). Under the agreement, the United States government provided assistance to help the government of Kazakhstan meet its healthcare goals, including healthcare reform and improvements in the quality of medical services (www.centralasia.usaid.gov; Amagoh 2011). In 2010, the United States Pharmacopeial Convention (USP) and *Kazakhstan's Republican State Enterprise (RSE)'s National Center for Expertise of Drugs, Medical Products and Equipment*, which is under the Ministry of Health, signed an agreement to share standards for the quality, purity, strength, and identity of medicines (Nafissa 2020).

8.3 Collaborations with the Private Sector (Public-Private-Partnerships)

Public–private partnerships (PPP) have helped governments address societal problems all over the world (Haque 2004; Klijn and Koppenjan 2016; Klijn and Teisman 2005). Public–private partnerships have been in the health sector globally with significant success (Sinisammal et al. 2016; Solheim-Kile and Wald 2020; Ungureanu et al. 2018; www.kppf.kz). The public–private partnership concept was first introduced in Kazakhstan in 2006. In an attempt to improve its legislative and institutional framework, and as part of *Salamaty*, Kazakhstan adopted the public–private partnership law in 2015, which created the basis for implementing public–private partnerships in almost all sectors, extended the list of public–private partnership participants and the forms and types of public–private partnership contracts, and introduced a private finance initiative (www.invest.com; Andrews et al. 2015; Klijn and Teisman 2003).

This has led to a significant increase in the number of public–private partnership projects implemented since 2016 (www.rcrz.kz; www.kppf.kz).

For example, while only 21 public–private partnership agreements were entered into in the period 2003–2016, 588 public–private partnership agreements were signed during the period January 2017 to February

2019. As of March 5, 2020, 1475 public–private partnership projects have been, or are in the process of being, implemented in Kazakhstan, of which approximately 20% are in the healthcare sector (Waheed et al. 2020).

Further improvements in the relevant legal framework have led to some amendments to the public–private partnership law, with the following results:

- Simplification of PPP planning through reduction in PPP project planning stages;
- Development of standard documentation with the aim of saving time for all parties involved; and
- The launch of a unified PPP database.

The *State Healthcare Development Program (Densaulyk) 2016–2019* enumerates several forms of cooperation between the public and private sectors, such as:

- Expanding participation of private medical providers in providing full range of services in guaranteed medical care and compulsory medical insurance;
- Transfer of some medical and non-medical services (such as, laboratories, radiological services, cleaning, food provision, maintenance of medical equipment, etc.) into long-term outsourcing;
- Attracting private firms to invest in the construction of healthcare facilities; and
- Involving private companies in the procurement of medical equipment, laboratory services, and IT systems in the healthcare sector. (Prime Minister of Kazakhstan 2019; Chaltabayeva 2020)

The *Program for Healthcare Development 2020–2025* provides a number of measures that encourage the government engagement with the private sector in the form of public–private partnerships (PPP) (www.lenta. inform.kz; www.pfie.com). These measures are aimed at facilitating the construction, modernization, and reconstruction of medical facilities and improving other areas of the healthcare system (Abdymanapov et al. 2016). The *Program for Healthcare Development 2020–2025* also provides mechanisms to improve the investment climate in the health sector through the adoption of corporate governance practices. It is estimated that 14 major PPP projects in the health sector will be implemented by 2027 (www.ppphealth4all.de).

8.4   Conclusion

Collaborations with other sectors and international organizations help to harness the expertise, skills, and funding needed to address the complex and challenging issues facing a healthcare system. Based on public sector reform perspective, Kazakhstan's health reforms encourage such partnerships in meeting the healthcare needs of the country. The government of Kazakhstan realizes that inputs from all entities, including civil society organizations, are needed in order to effectively address the country's healthcare challenges. Significant improvements have been made in the health system in terms of infrastructure development, procurement of advanced medical technologies, and the training and competence of healthcare workers. Further health reforms in the future are expected to strengthen such partnerships and collaborations with more benefits for Kazakhstan's healthcare system.

References

Abdymanapov, S., Toxanova, A., Galiyeva, A., Abildina, A., and Aitkaliyeva, A. (2016). Development of public-private partnership in the Republic of Kazakhstan. *IEJME-Mathematical Education,* Vol. 11 No. 5, pp. 1113–1126.

Adams, J., and Garbutt, A. (2008). Participatory monitoring and evaluation in practice: lessons from Central Asia. INTRAC, *Praxis Paper* 21.

Alymkulova, A., and Seipulnick, D. (2005). NGO strategy for survival in Central Asia: financial sustainability. *The William Davidson Institute, Policy Brief,* No. 22.

Amagoh, F. (2011). New public management and healthcare reform in Kazakhstan. *International Journal of Public Administration,* Vol. 34 No. 9, 567–578.

Andrews, R., Esteve, M. and Ysa, T. (2015). Public–private joint ventures: mixing oil and water? *Public Money and Management,* Vol. 35 No. 4, pp. 265–272.

Bergamaschi, I., Moore, P., and Tickner, A. (2017). *South-South Cooperation Beyond the Myths: Rising Donors, New Aid Practices?* Palgrave Macmillan.

Brinkerhoff, D. (2002). Government-nonprofit partners for health sector reform in Central Asia: family group practitioners in Kazakhstan and Kyrgyzstan. *Public Administration and Development,* Vol. 22 No. 1, 51–61.

Buxton, C. (2009). NGO networks in Central Asia and global civil society: potentials and limitations. *Central Asian Survey,* Vol. 28 No. 1, pp. 43–58.

Chaltabayeva, R. (2020). PPP in healthcare: critical issues, best practice and Kazakh realities. (available at: https://www.unicaselaw.com/storage/app/uploads/public/5e5/f87/5ba/5e5f875ba941e432245942.pdf).

Civil Alliance of Kazakhstan (2011). *Non-governmental Organizations of Kazakhstan: 20 years of development.* Almaty, Kazakhstan: Civil Alliance of Kazakhstan.

Diachenko, S. (2008). *The Government and NGOs in Kazakhstan: Strategy, Forms, and Mechanisms of Cooperation.* CA & CC Press, Sweden.

GerstIberger, W. and Schneider, K. (2013). Outsourcing and concession models as door opener for public-private partnerships in the European health sector? *International Journal of Public Sector Management,* Vol. 26 No. 7, pp. 554–575.

Haque, M. (2004). Government based on partnership with NGOs: implications for development and empowerment in rural Bangladesh. *International Review of Administrative Sciences,* Vol. 70 N0. 2, pp. 271–290.

Kabdiyeva, A., and Dixon, J. (2014). Collaboration between the state and NGOs in Kazakhstan. *International Journal of Community and Cooperative Studies,* Vol. 1 No. 2, pp. 27–41.

Kazakhstan (2006). Concept of civil society development in Kazakhstan for 2006–2011. (Available at: http://npoastana.kz//library..).

Klijn, E. and Koppenjan, J. (2016). The impact of contract characteristics on the performance of public–private partnerships (PPPs). *Public Money and Management,* Vol. 36 No. 6, pp. 455–462.

Klijn, E. and Teisman, G. (2003). Institutional and strategic barriers to public-private-partnership: an analysis of Dutch cases. *Public Money and Management,* Vol. 23 No. 3, pp. 137–146.

Klijn, E. and Teisman, G. (2005). Public-private partnerships as the management of co-production: strategic and institutional obstacles in a difficult marriage. In Hodge, G. and Greve, C. (Eds), *The Challenge of Public-Private Partnerships: Learning from International Experience,* Edward Elgar, Cheltenham, pp. 95–116.

Katsaga, A., Kulzhanov, M., Karanikolos, M., and Rechel, B. (2012). Kazakhstan: Health system overview. *In Health systems in Transition,* Karanikolos M. and Rechel, B. (eds.), Geneva: European Observatory on Health Systems and Policies.

www.kppf.kz. PPP projects: construction and operation of a multi-profile university hospital for 300 beds in the city of Karaganda. (available at: https://kppf.kz/en/news/gchp/133).

Kulzhanov, M., and Rechel, B. (2007). Kazakhstan: health system overview. *In Health systems in Transition,* B. Rechel (Ed.), Geneva: European Observatory on Health Systems and Policies.

www.lenta.inform.kz. Kazakhstan to build 20 multi-field hospitals by 2020 through PPP. (available at: https://www.lenta.inform.kz/en/kazakhstan-to-build-20-multi-field-hospitals-by-2025-through-ppp_a3689860).

Makhmutova, M. and Akhmetova, A. (2011). *Civil Society in Kazakhstan,* Almaty, Kazakhstan: Civicus.

Ministry of Health of the Republic of Kazakhstan (2002). *Health of population and health care of Republic of Kazakhstan, 1991–2001.* Astana, Ministry of Health.

Ministry of Health of the Republic of Kazakhstan (2004). National Program of Healthcare Reform and Development for 2005–2010, *approved by presidential decree on 13 September, 2004.* Astana, Ministry of Health.

Ministry of National Economy of the Republic of Kazakhstan: Statistics Committee. (2018). *Statistics of Foreign and Mutual Aid.*

Nafissa, I. (2020). On becoming a development cooperation partner: Kazakhstan's foreign policy, identity, and international norms. *Journal of Eurasian Studies,* Vol. 11 No. 2, pp. 158–173.

Ovcharenko, V. (2004). The state-civil society relationship in Kazakhstan: mechanisms of cooperation and support. *The International Journal Not-for-Profit Law,* 6, 3. (retrieved from: http://www.icnl.org/knowledge/ijnl/vol6iss3/art_4.htm).

www.pfie.com. Kazakhstan's health PPP program. (available at: https://www.pfie.com/story/2368789/kazakhstans-health-ppp-programme-l8n2d267f).

President of Kazakhstan (1997). *Kazakhstan 2030: Prosperity, Security and Welfare for all People of Kazakhstan.* Almaty, President of the Republic of Kazakhstan.

President of Kazakhstan (1998). *The Health of the Nation,* Almaty, President of Republic of Kazakhstan.

Prime Minister of Kazakhstan. (2019). *Emphasis on Healthy Lifestyles and Human Capital: About the Program of Healthcare Development 2020–2025.* Nur-Sultan, Kazakhstan.

www.ppphealth4all.de. Kazakhstan: hospitals modernization program in healthcare – planning advisory services for PPP projects. (available at: https://ppphealth4all.de/kazakhstan-hospitals-modernisation-programme-healthcare-planning-advisory-services-for-ppp-projects).

www.rcrz.kz. Public-private partnership (PPP) projects in healthcare. (available at: http://www.rcrz.kz/index.php/en/for-chiefs/public-private-partnership).

Sinisammal, J., Leviakkangas, P. Autio, T. and Hyrkas, E. (2016). Entrepreneurs' perspective on public-private partnership in health care and social services. *Journal of Health Organization and Management,* Vol. 30 No. 1, pp. 174–191

Solheim-Kile, E. and Wald, Andreas (2020). Public-private joint ventures in the healthcare sector: enlarging the shadow of the future through social and economic incentives. *International Journal of Public Sector Management,* (online first) doi: https://doi.org/10.1108/IJPS-12-20190318.

Ungureanu, P., Bertolotti, F. and Macri, D. (2018). Brokers or platforms? A longitudinal study of how hybrid inter-organizational partnerships for regional innovation deal with VUCA environments. *European Journal of Innovation Management,* Vol. 21 No. 4, pp. 636–671.

Waheed, A., Bakenova, A. and Zhumakhanov, D. (2020). Kazakhstan's health PPP program. (available at: https://www.morganlewis.com/-/media/files/

publication/outside-publication/article/2020/kazakhstans-health-ppp-programme.pdf).

World Bank (2007). *World Development Indicators*. Washington, DC, World Bank.

World Bank. (2012). *WDI – World Development Indicators*. World Bank.

CHAPTER 9

Future Prospects and Conclusion

In more than three decades, Kazakhstan has made significant efforts to reform its healthcare system. Several reform programs were undertaken, starting from *Concept on Healthcare Reform* in 1992. The main aims of the health reforms have been to modernize the health system in line with western best practices, and provide quality healthcare to the population in a cost-effective manner. The analysis shows that Kazakhstan embarked on an approach that focuses on a process of "continuous improvement" in reforming its healthcare system by periodically upgrading and modernizing the system every few years. In analyzing healthcare reforms in Kazakhstan, this book has examined several parts of the reforms within the context of public sector reform paradigm. Public sector reform comprises of mechanisms and processes through which governments engage other sectors (private, and non-governmental organizations) to deliver public goods and services innovatively and cost-effectively without sacrificing quality. Public sector reform is built on the ideas of New Public Management (NPM) and New Public Governance (NPG) (Analoui 2009; Devlin 2010; Howe 2012; Pedersen and Rendtorff 2010). Consequently, this book analyzes Kazakhstan's health reform policies through the following prisms of public sector reform: decentralization; efficiency; quality; human resources; competition; and partnerships and collaborative arrangements.

Decentralization is associated with improved service delivery in Kazakhstan. Decentralization empowers local bodies to make policy decisions on behalf of their communities (Jones et al. 2013; Liou 2007;

F. E. Amagoh, *Healthcare Policies in Kazakhstan*,
https://doi.org/10.1007/978-981-16-2370-7_9

Panjaitan et al. 2019). The decentralization efforts in Kazakhstan's health sector have been achieved mostly through the privatization of facilities and the devolution of administrative and financial responsibilities from national level to *oblast*, and to a very limited extent *rayon* levels (Ministry of Health of the Republic of Kazakhstan 2004; Amagoh 2011; Katsaga et al. 2012). The health reforms have gradually given regional and local authorities more roles and responsibilities in the delivery of healthcare services to the population.

Several measures that have been put in place to improve efficiency through the health reforms and there have been significant improvements in the reduction of redundancies in the health system, less reliance on inpatient care, and a focus on primary healthcare. The reforms have also led to more focus on disease prevention and healthy lifestyles which will lead to significant cost-savings in the long-run. The gaps in regional inequities have been considerably reduced (OECD 2018; Committee on Statistics, Ministry of the National Economy of the Republic of Kazakhstan 2016).

Quality improvement measures constitute perhaps some of the most notable outcomes of the health reform efforts. The reforms have led to improved health quality through the adoption of international standards of quality and performance indicators. Measures have been put in place to ensure that healthcare professionals have the requisite professional skills and education needed to pass international medical certification examinations. A competitive environment has been created by encouraging private medical practice and providing free choice of doctors and medical facilities for citizens.

Inter-sectoral collaborations with the private sector and non-governmental organizations, as well as engagements with international organizations and donor agencies have brought in much-needed expertise and funds for the modernization of the health system. The reforms, through these collaborative arrangements, initiated major changes to healthcare provision and governance.

Outcomes of Kazakhstan's health reform programs show a trend of steady improvements in health indicators over the years. This can be seen in the progression of positive health outcomes the country has achieved since independence. For example, as explained earlier, in Table 1.4 while life expectancy was 68.3 years in 1990, it increased to 73.9 years in 2020 (Table 1.4). Infant mortality reduced from 51.4 deaths (per 1000 live births) in 1990 to 9.2 deaths (per 1000 live births) in 2018. Similarly, maternal mortality reduced from 78 deaths (per 1000 live births) in 1990 to 10 deaths (per 1000 live births) in 2016 (the latest available data). These are significant achievements that arguably would not have been realized without the concerted efforts of the government to improve the health standards of the population through the continuous improvements of the health system and the reform programs. Other indicators, such as death rate (per 1000 population), under-5 year mortality (per 1000 live births), and so on follow the same positive trajectory.

Finally, Kazakhstan's *Health Care Index* improved from a ranking of 88th position in 2020 to a ranking of 58th position in 2021 (www.nubeo. com). The *Health Care Index* is an estimate of the overall quality of a country's healthcare system, healthcare professionals, technologies, costs, and so on. Kazakhstan is the only Central Asian country included in the ranking. However, Kazakhstan's ranking in 2021 surpassed that of Russia (60th position), Belarus (90th position), Ukraine (79th position), and Azerbaijan (91st position). These indicators show that the efforts of Kazakhstan's government are yielding sustainable long-term positive results.

9.1   FUTURE OUTLOOK AND PANDEMIC RESPONSE STRATEGIES

As Kazakhstan looks toward the future, plans are already in place to further upgrade the health system through additional reforms as part of the *Kazakhstan 2050 Strategy* which aims to make Kazakhstan among the 30 most developed economies in the world by 2050 (www.kfm.gov.kz).

Efforts are being made to improve the country's human capital through, amongst other things, significant investments in the health infrastructure and continuous innovation in healthcare delivery (www.covid19healthsystem.gov). The COVID-19 outbreak has affected the global community, such that even the most advanced countries were not prepared to deal with such an outbreak. Significantly, the COVID-19 pandemic has been a test case on the impacts of the reforms on the Kazakh health system. It has shown what lessons can be learned from government response strategies, and how such lessons can be included in future health reforms in the Kazakhstan.

The COVID-19 outbreak has shown the vulnerability of health systems around the world to pandemic health situations. The global community and the WHO have made efforts to contain the virus and mitigate its impacts on global health.

A comprehensive mix of policies, with emphasis on testing, tracing and isolation, mask-wearing, and social distancing offer the best hope to limiting the lockdown and containing the spread of the virus (OECD 2020).

A prominent tool to track governments' responses to the COVID-19 pandemic is the *Oxford's Coronavirus Government Response Tracker (OxCGRT)* (also known as *COVI-19 Tracker*) (www.en.unesco.org).

The *COVID-19 Tracker* uses data from countries around the world to assess governments' containment and closure policies (such as school closures and restrictions in movement); economic policies; and health policies (such as testing regimes) (https://ourworldindata.org/). The measure calculates *Government Response Stringency Index.* The *Government Response Stringency Index* is based on a score of 0–100. A higher score means a stricter government response (that is, 0 = weakest response, and 100 = strictest response) (www.covidtracker.bsg). The index is calculated based on 9 metrics which consist of the following (www.data.humdata.org):

- School closures;
- Workplace closures;
- Cancellation of public events;
- Restrictions of public gatherings;
- Closure of public transport;
- Stay-at-home requirements;
- Public information campaigns;
- Restrictions of internal movements; and
- international travel controls.

The Index changes on a daily basis based on governments' response strategies. For example, an examination of the Index for Central Asian countries from December 25, 2020, to January 25, 2021, shows that Kazakhstan's *Government Response Stringency Index* was 75.0 on December 25, 2020, and 68.52 on January 23, 2021. This is in line with top performers in the *Stringency Response Index* among Central Asian countries, such as Uzbekistan and Kyrgyzstan as shown in Table 9.1. These *Government Response Stringency Index* scores for Kazakhstan indicate a relatively modest response to the COVID-19 pandemic.

While it is true that global coordination on public responses is needed to control such a pandemic, it is also important to have domestic as well as regional containment policies. Thus, measures to control COVID-19

Table 9.1 COVID-19 Government Response Stringency Index for CIS Countries

	March 25, 2020	April 25, 2020	May 25, 2020	June 25, 2020	July 25, 2020	August 25, 2020	Sep. 25, 2020	Oct. 25, 2020	Nov. 25, 2020	Dec. 25, 2020	Jan. 22, 2020
Kazakhstan	**80.09**	**92.13**	**83.80**	**81.02**	**83.33**	**79.63**	**78.70**	**74.07**	**66.20**	**75.00**	**68.52**
Kyrgyzstan	92.13	92.13	79.17	76.61	76.39	73.61	67.13	55.09	53.25	49.07	41.67
Tajikistan	19.44	40.74	44.44	65.74	49.07	47.22	33.33	36.11	33.33	38.89	44.44
Turkmenistan	50.93	31.48	31.48	28.70	47.22	47.22	47.22	63.89	63.89	55.56	–
Uzbekistan	80.56	90.74	86.11	66.20	71.30	51.85	43.52	39.81	39.81	42.59	46.30

Source: Our World in data (www.ourworldindata.org)

must include local risk assessments. This means that if an outbreak occurs, it must be limited to the local level with targeted movement restrictions in accordance with national recommendations. To this end, Kazakhstan launched a mobile app *("Saqbol")* with the aim of controlling the spread of the virus and quickly localizing the spots of infection (www.egov.kz). To mitigate the spread of the virus, Kazakhstan promoted public health measures, invested in hospital surge capacities, repurposed some hospitals, and built new hospitals.

9.2   Conclusion

This book has presented the health reform programs that Kazakhstan's government is using to modernize its health system within the perspective of public sector reform. The discussion, analysis, and health indicators in Kazakhstan show the positive impacts of the reforms on the lives the population. The importance of well-optimized and robust health policies in reducing diseases and deaths and improving human well-being cannot be over-emphasized. Reforms of health systems have the potential to enhance human capital and national development. Limited resources available to governments mean that it has to take serious commitment to prioritize continuous improvements of the health system through incremental reforms in order to meet the health needs of the populations. Kazakhstan has proven that having a consistent and continuous improvement strategy which uses health reform policies constitutes one of the best approaches to address a country's healthcare challenges. Going forward, and with new experiences gained from the COVID-19 pandemic, subsequent health reform policies should explore how Kazakhstan can be better prepared to address such health emergencies in the future.

References

Amagoh, F. (2011). New public management and healthcare reform in Kazakhstan. *International Journal of Public Administration, 34,* 9, 567–578.

Analoui, F. (2009). Challenges of successful reform: an international perspective. *Journal of Management Development,* Vol. 28 No. 6, pp. 489–494.

Committee on Statistics, Ministry of the National Economy of the Republic of Kazakhstan. (2016). *Socio-economic development of the Republic of Kazakhstan,* Astana.

www.covidtracker.bsg. Oxford COVID-19 Government Response Tracker (available at: https://covidtracker.bsg.ox.ac.uk/).

www.covid19healthsystem.gov. Policy responses for Kazakhstan. (available at: https://www.covid19healthsystem.org/countries/kazakhstan/livinghit. aspx?Section=5.%20Governance&Type=Chapter).

www.data.humdata.org. Oxford COVID-19 Government Response Stringency Index (available at: https://data.humdata.org/dataset/oxford-covid-19-government-response-tracker).

Devlin, P. (2010). Exploring efficiency's dominance: the wholeness of the process. *Quantitative Research in Accounting and Management,* Vol. 7 No. 2, pp. 141–162.

www.egov.kz. Saqbol mobile app. (available at: http://egov.kz/cms/en/information/about/Saqbol_mobileapp).

www.en.unesco.org. Oxford Covid-19 government response tracker: systematic information on government measures. (available at: https://en.unesco.org/inclusivepolicylab/learning/oxford-covid-19-government-response-tracker).

Howe, B. (2012). Governance in the interest of the most vulnerable. *Public Admin. Dev.,* Vol. 32 Nos 4–5, pp. 345–356.

Jones, S., Aryal, K. and Collins, A. (2013). Local-level governance of risk and resilience in Nepal. *Disasters,* Vol. 37 No. 3, pp. 442–467.

Katsaga, A., Kulzhanov, M., Karanikolos, M., and Rechel, B. (2012). Kazakhstan: Health system overview. *In Health systems in Transition,* Karanikolos M. and Rechel, B. (eds.), Geneva: European Observatory on Health Systems and Policies.

www.kfm.gov.kz. *Kazakhstan 2050 Strategy.* (available at: https://kfm.gov.kz/en/activity/strategy-and-program/strategy-kazakhstan-2050/).

Liou, K. (2007). Applying good governance concept to promote local economic development: Contribution and challenges. *International Journal of Economic Development,* Vol. 9, No. 1/2, pp. 1–31.

Ministry of Health of the Republic of Kazakhstan (2004). National Program of Health Reform and Development for 2005–2010, *approved by presidential decree on 13 September, 2004.* Astana, Ministry of Health.

OECD. (2020). Walking the tightrope: avoiding a lockdown while containing the virus. In *OECD: Tackling Coronavirus (COVID-19): Contributing to a Global Effort.* OECD Publishing, Paris.

OECD (2018), *OECD Reviews of Health Systems: Kazakhstan.* OECD Publishing, Paris

www.ourworldindata.org. COVID-19: government stringency index, January 25, 2021. (available at: https://ourworldindata.org/grapher/covid-stringency-index).

Panjaitan, R., Sarwono, S., and Saleh, C. (2019). "The role of central government and local government and the moderating effect of good governance on forest fire policy in Indonesia", *Benchmarking: An International Journal*, Vol. 26 No. 1, pp. 147–159.

Pedersen, J. and Rendtorff, J. (2010). Balancing values and economic efficiency in the public sector: what can public welfare service institutions learn from private service firms? *Social and Business Review*, Vol. 5 No. 3, pp. 293–302.

INDEX